Small Animal Fracture Repair
A Case-Based Approach

Karl H. Kraus
DVM, MS, Professor and Section Head,
Small Animal Surgery, Veterinary Clinical Sciences,
College of Veterinary Medicine, Iowa State University, USA

Steven M. Fox
MS, DVM, MBA, PhD, President of Fox Third Bearing Inc,
President Securos Surgical, Adjunct Associate Professor, Massey University (NZ),
Adjunct Assistant Professor at the University of Illinois,
Advisor to the University of Tennessee Pain Center, USA

Fredrick S. Pike
DVM, DACVS, Staff Surgeon, Managing Medical Director,
Veterinary Specialty Hospital, San Diego, USA

Emily C. Salzer
Veterinary Clinical Sciences, College of Veterinary Medicine,
Iowa State University, USA

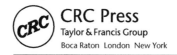

CRC Press
Taylor & Francis Group
Boca Raton London New York

CRC Press is an imprint of the
Taylor & Francis Group, an **informa** business

CRC Press
Taylor & Francis Group
6000 Broken Sound Parkway NW, Suite 300
Boca Raton, FL 33487-2742

First issued in paperback 2020

© 2017 by Taylor & Francis Group, LLC
CRC Press is an imprint of Taylor & Francis Group, an Informa business

No claim to original U.S. Government works

ISBN 13: 978-0-367-57443-7 (pbk)
ISBN 13: 978-1-4987-3242-0 (hbk)

Visit the Taylor & Francis Web site at
http://www.taylorandfrancis.com

and the CRC Press Web site at
http://www.crcpress.com

Contents

Part 1   Basic Concepts

Part 2   Clinical Cases

Contributors of Case Material

Please note that some contributors were residents during the clinical cases detailed.

Anthony E. Acquaviva, VMD, DACVS-SA

Sean Aiken, DVM, MS, DACVS-SA

Ben J. Bayer, DVM, DACVS-SA

Mary Sarah Bergh, DVM, DACVS-SA

Andrew Burton, DVM, DACVS-SA

William Hoefle, DVM, DACVS

Jennifer L. Huck, DVM, DACVS-SA

Joshua Jackson, DVM, DACVS-SA

Nina Kieves, DVM, DACVS-SA

Alexander Krebs, DVM, DACVS-SA

Emily I. Miller, DVM, DACVS-SA

Megan Templeton, DVM, DACVS-SA

Angel M. Thompson, DVM, DACVS-SA

Eric Zellner, DVM

Preface

Fracture cases can be dramatic and intimidating. Dramatic, as they are often caused by motor vehicle accidents or other trauma. The patient can be in shock with other concomitant injuries. There are often deformities of the limb(s), debilitation and pain. Intimidating, because they are infrequent in most primary practices. Fractures can vary widely in severity and complexity. There are many different, and ostensibly complex, fixation devices available. Mistakes and failures are glaringly obvious on radiographs. There are usually a number of opinions amongst surgeons as to the best way to treat a specific fracture. The end result is that a student, practitioner, or even experienced surgeon may have doubts about the best way to handle a specific patient's fracture(s).

The intention of this book is to provide some small degree of guidance to the understanding and treatment of fracture cases. This book consists of two parts. Part I is a very concise overview of fracture biology and mechanics, including the use and 'rules' of various basic orthopedic devices. This part is not intended to be a complete or exhaustive treatise on fracture repair. There are many available texts on veterinary surgery and fracture repair and the reader should refer to these for more in-depth discussion. Part I presents some basic concepts that support those clinical decisions presented in Part II.

Part II is an anthology of cases demonstrating successful treatments for more common fractures seen in small animal veterinary practice. Each case starts with pertinent history and physical examination findings, patient assessment, fracture description and assessment, and options for fracture repair methods. The surgery report follows with a step-by-step approach to the surgical procedure, including some 'tips and tricks' to performing the fracture repair successfully. The postoperative radiographs are then assessed using the four 'A's': Alignment, Apposition, Apparatus and Activity (for follow-up assessment).

It has been a long-standing frustration for the authors to read and hear of cases reported to 'do fine' postoperatively without the support of follow-up radiographs. Not all fracture healing is elegant, as is witnessed by the following inclusive cases. A fracture having healed with a large and ugly callus can be an absolute clinical success. Each case within this text has at least one follow-up set of radiographs, and each case was considered to have had a successful outcome; the animal returning to activity following the last set of radiographs presented and the owner's expectations having been met.

This text is meant to be helpful on several different levels. First, for the veterinary student this is a quick and highly visual reference of many different types of fractures and repair techniques to aid in the understanding of osteosynthesis. Second, for the practitioner who performs little, or no, orthopedic surgery, this book will serve as a quick reference guide. They can compare their own case to one or more of the examples in Part II of the text. Insights gained from these cases can assist the practitioner when advising pet owners of the methods an orthopedic surgeon may recommend and will help the primary care provider communicate with a referring surgeon. Those in the early stage of their surgical career will find Parts I and II a helpful guide in decision making and surgical technique. For the 'seasoned' orthopedist, the cases presented may either reinforce or offer new alternatives with regard to techniques and devices they commonly favor.

Of course there is a broad spectrum of fracture configurations and levels of complexity, and many different opinions regarding the 'best method' of repair for each fracture. We fully acknowledge that there is more than one way to repair many, if not most, fractures. As much as is practical, examples of different approaches and devices are presented within the limits of our available case materials. We also have our biases regarding fixation selections, and the authors, as well as some contributors, have direct or indirect financial interests in some of the devices presented. With successive editions, we hope to broaden the number of case contributors, therein also broadening our collective insight from 'thinking outside the box'.

These surgeons were attending clinicians and primary or assisting surgeons on the cases in Part II.

We hope that you find this text helpful in assessing, triaging, and operating fracture cases for the benefit of our patients.

'A House is Not a Home Without a Dog'

Karl H. Kraus, DVM, MS, Dipl. ACVS
Steven M. Fox, MS, DVM, MBA PhD
Fredrick S. Pike, DVM, Dipl. ACVS-SA
Emily C. Salzer, DVM

Acknowledgements

We would like to thank our colleagues who keep us sharp, the animal owners that allow us to do what we love, our families who keep us happy, and our patients whose amazing capacity to heal makes us look good.

List of Abbreviations

AMI   Area Moment of Inertia
DCP   Dynamic Compression Plate
IM   Intramedullary (pinning)
J   Joule
LC-DCP   Limited Contact Dynamic Compression Plate
MIPO   Minimally Invasive Plate Osteosynthesis
PRP   Platelet Rich Plasma
SOP   String of Pearls
TPLO   Tibial Plateau Leveling Osteotomy

Measurement Units

Please note that apparatus dimensions are provided in centimeters (cm) or millimeters (mm). Wire diameters are provided in millimeters and US wire gauge.

Part 1

Basic Concepts

Patient and Fracture Assessment

The goals for surgical treatment of fractures (osteosynthesis) are as follows.

- Union of the fracture as a functional anatomical and mechanical structure.
- Appropriate healing of soft tissues.
- Return to function of the limb.

Fundamentals of Tissue Healing

Mechanisms of tissue healing are important and a thorough understanding of wound and fracture healing dictate treatment choices as well as implant selection; only a brief overview is included.

The three phases of wound healing are as follows.

1. Inflammatory
2. Fibroblastic (proliferative)
3. Remodeling (maturation)

The inflammatory phase typically lasts up to four days post trauma and the magnitude of the inflammatory phase is related to the magnitude of trauma. The fibroblastic phase begins at three-to-four days with the removal of debris and infiltration of granulation tissue. Infiltrative granulation tissue contains fibroblasts; myofibroblasts, pericytes and endothelial cells which regenerate capillaries and larger vessels, in addition to keratinocytes for epithelialization. The inflammatory phase of healing can span several days to two or more weeks for soft tissue damage compared with several months for bone. This results in varying amounts of reparative tissue being formed depending on the biological and mechanical environment. Once the basic integrity of the healing wound is formed, either bone or soft tissue, then remodeling, or maturation, commences. The remodeling/maturation phase can take several months to several years, as the body attempts to re-establish anatomical form and function of the damaged tissues.

Bone Healing

Bone healing occurs via two different mechanisms: primary and secondary bone healing.[1] Primary bone healing follows anatomic alignment of fracture fragments and rigid anatomic reduction, often with interfragmentary compression. Bone fragment contact (contact healing), or gaps less than 1 mm between cortical bone fragments (gap healing), are critical for primary bone healing. Small gaps are filled with bone perpendicular to the long axis of the bone or along fracture lines. New bone is directly formed through osteoclasts crossing the fracture gaps or lines, followed by osteoblasts transitioning to osteocytes, which subsequently form new bone matrices and establish a lamellar architecture (Haversian system). The remodeling cellular units are often called 'cutting cones'. Secondary bone healing occurs in fracture gaps and/or where there is motion between fracture fragments. In these cases, new bone forms by cells transitioning through granulation to cartilage which is then converted to bone by the process of endochondral ossification. The composite of cells formed (which includes newly formed cartilage and bone) is called a callus. The size of the callus that forms is contingent on blood supply, motion, and age of the patient (Figure 1.1). Callus is then converted to lamellar bone by cellular units (cutting cones) using mechanisms similar to primary bone healing.

Tissue Healing Considerations

Volumes have been previously written on the mechanisms of soft tissue and bone healing.[2–4] However, these can be condensed to a set of basic considerations when assessing your patient and their fracture. The patient should be thoroughly evaluated with expected healing in mind. High-energy wounds result in marked soft tissue damage and heal with a more robust and longer inflammatory phase. If permissible, surgical intervention should be staged, with first attention to the soft tissue trauma. Soft tissue wounds may heal following a more exuberant fibroblastic phase. This would be welcome in situations enhanced by a large callus, but not so if the fibrous response compromises muscle, tendon or joint function. Insufficient attention to accompanying soft tissue trauma may give rise to retarded bone healing due to a compromised blood supply for tissue healing support.

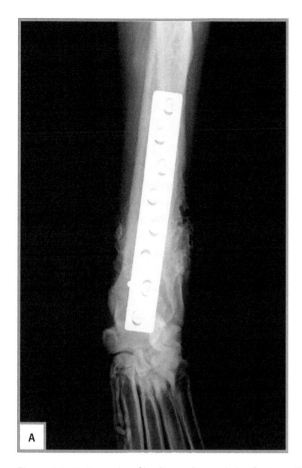

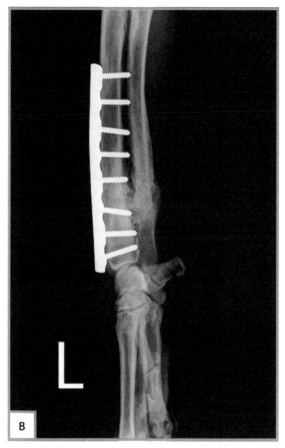

Figure 1.1 Radiographs of healing radius and ulna fractures illustrating callus formation. (A) postoperative: cranial/caudal view; (B) postoperative: lateral view. Plate osteosynthesis was performed with a DCP to allow dynamic compression. Note that the screws are located eccentrically away from the fracture line so that weight-bearing causes compression across the transverse fracture. The ulna was not repaired. The radius healed through primary bone union with minimal callus. The ulna healed with callus formation and is undergoing endochondral ossification.

The type of bone healing that is desired (primary or secondary) needs early consideration. Joint fractures should be rigidly and anatomically repaired (striving for primary bone union), so that callus or incongruity does not lead to a decreased range of motion and osteoarthritis. Areas of scant soft tissue coverage of bone or minimal endosteal blood supply are less likely to heal with secondary bone union, and should therefore be treated using techniques that encourage primary bone union. The treatment of distal radius and ulna fractures in small dogs are classic examples of when dynamic compression plating is preferential to buttress plating or external fixation.[5] This is primarily due to the simple fracture configurations and the limited blood supply of this anatomical location. Interfragmentary compression can be achieved in these cases but the limited blood supply may be insufficient for secondary bone union.

Secondary bone union occurs most readily in specific fractures. For example, femoral, humeral, and pelvic fractures heal well by secondary bone union because of the abundant soft tissue coverage and robust blood supply. For these types of fracture, buttress plating with locking plates is often the treatment choice. Metaphyseal bone, which has rich vascularization, heals well by secondary bone healing. However, some fractures must heal by secondary bone union as anatomic alignment is not possible to allow primary bone union. Trying to anatomically reconstruct a highly comminuted femoral fracture, for example, frequently compromises normal healing mechanisms. This delays osteosynthesis and has an accompanying increased chance of infection and non-union.[6]

Patient Considerations

Age is a major consideration when evaluating the fracture patient.[7] Juvenile bone heals much faster than adult bone, and geriatric patient bone can have delayed healing. If slower healing is anticipated, more rigid implants with a longer functional activity may be preferred. Ancillary procedures such as augmentation with bone grafting, cytokines, stem cells or platelet rich plasma (PRP) may be beneficial. Juvenile bone can also be softer than adult bone. Implants and devices that are weakly anchored in soft bone are less suitable than stronger constructs; locking screw plates and external fixators are often preferential to dynamic compression plates, for this reason.[8, 9]

Debilitated, often older, patients typically require more attentive treatment than younger, healthy patients. Specific attention should be given to appropriate nutrition and concomitant treatment of any pre-existing disease. Be aware however, that older patients tend to recover more quickly at home and all efforts should be made to discharge them from the hospital as soon as possible.

Patient size affects many aspects of bone healing, specifically in very large or very small patients. Very large patients may be too large for standard implants available for fracture repair in smaller-sized animals. For example, it would be inappropriate to use a 3.5 mm dynamic compression plate (DCP) for a tibia fracture in a dog weighing 100 kg, when the plate is used in buttress. Likewise, if a patient is very small it is tempting to use implants that are proportional. Remember that the area moment of inertia (AMI) for implants reflects non-linear increases in strength and stiffness as the dimensions of the implant increase. Surgeons often choose a screw or external fixator pin that is no greater than 20 percent of the bone diameter. As animals increase in size, their bones become relatively larger in linear proportion to their size and weight. However, the stiffness of increasingly larger

implants is dictated by the AMI; which for a rod, is the radius to the fourth power (r^4). Accordingly, the relative strength of an implant becomes greater as the implant becomes larger. Conversely, very small patients will require small implants and these are geometrically less stiff and weaker. As a consequence, comparatively larger implants may need to be chosen for smaller patients in order to achieve the same relative stiffness.

The normal activity levels of the patient should also be considered. More passive/docile patients will not place as much demand on fixation constructs as very active patients. Some young, active animals can 'over-ride' their concomitant physiologic pain to the detriment of their fixation repair. Again, these patients may have an anticipated need for a more robust fixation. Also, if they are very active or aggressive, constructs such as external fixators, that require frequent attention, may not be recommended or should be used with caution.

Owner Considerations

There are several owner considerations before determining a type of fracture repair. First, some owners are more compliant than others regarding patient care instructions. This includes exercise restriction as well as medications. A caregiver that is unable to closely monitor and care for their patient is less likely, for example, to accommodate an external fixator so internal fixation techniques should be favored. Additionally, appropriate routes of pain medication or antibiotics, with less frequent dosing intervals, would be more sensible.

Second, finance is often a significant issue for owners unexpectedly faced with a pet's injury requiring surgery. The cost of implants vary and some implant costs are prohibitive. Although cost should not dictate repair technique, there are occasions when a simpler, less costly method can be successful even if not the optimal choice. For example, a pin and wire fixation of a spiral oblique tibial fracture is a fraction of the implant cost of a lag screw and locking plate repair.

Third, owner expectations need to be considered. For some performance animals, a return to full athletic function is desired. Other clients have less demanding expectations and will accept less than full function or some amount of disability. An excellent outcome for all repairs is unrealistic.

There may be permanent impairment of function and ultimately amputation may result in a better quality of life for the patient.

Fracture Assessment Implications for Healing and Implant Choice

First the surgeon should carefully assess the fracture by completing radiographic views, and a visual inspection and palpation of the fracture. Any assessment is performed systematically with consideration of the following.

1. Assessing if the fracture is open or closed.
2. Determining characteristics of the bone fracture and capacity for healing.
3. Extent of the fracture within the bone (and joint).
4. Kinetic energy associated with both the fractured bone and soft tissue damage.
5. Evaluation of soft tissue coverage and soft tissue viability.
6. Fracture displacement.
7. Length of time from fracture occurrence to anticipated repair.
8. General health of the patient.

The most commonly used classification system for open fractures is the Gustilo-Anderson classification.[10, 11] This system aids prognosis of infection, non-union and other complication rates. It also provides a guide to treatment, antibiotic

recommendations, timing for interventions and surgery. It enables a quick, consistent communication system for surgeons and researchers. Classification of fracture severity reflects the amount of energy, extent of soft tissue injury and the extent of contamination. Open fractures are classified as grades I–III. Open, grade III fractures are sub-classified as A, B, or C (see Table 1.1).

Although the classification system is helpful in communicating the severity of open fractures and generally dictating treatment, it is not very specific and clinicians are often in disagreement. Specifically the system does not clearly indicate the amount of energy imparted, nor any neurological damage or the degree of vascular compromise.

Grade I or II open fractures, when treated early, have little effect on prognosis or treatment choices. Treatment includes early and aggressive antibiotic treatment with a broad spectrum antibiotic. This is usually a first generation cephalosporin which should be administered as soon as possible parenterally and at the highest end of therapeutic

Table 1.1 Grade classification and sub-classification for open fractures

Grade	Description
I	Open fracture, clean wound, wound <1 cm in length.
II	Open fracture, wound >1 cm but <10 cm, without extensive soft tissue damage, flaps, avulsions.
III	Open with extensive soft-tissue laceration >10 cm, damage or loss or an open segmental fracture. Fractures requiring vascular repair, or open fractures untreated for over 8 hours.
Sub-classification of open grade III fractures	
IIIA	Type III fracture with adequate periosteal coverage of the fracture bone despite extensive soft tissue damage.
IIIB	Type III fracture with extensive soft tissue loss, periosteal stripping and bone damage. Massive contamination, need for soft tissue coverage procedure (flaps). An example of this type of fracture is seen in Figure 1.2.
IIIC	Type III fracture associated with arterial injury requiring vascular repair.

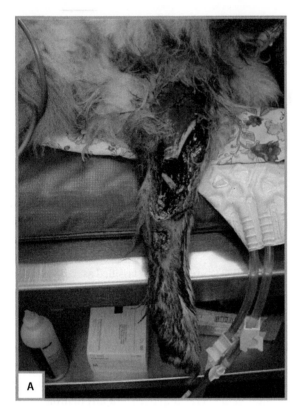
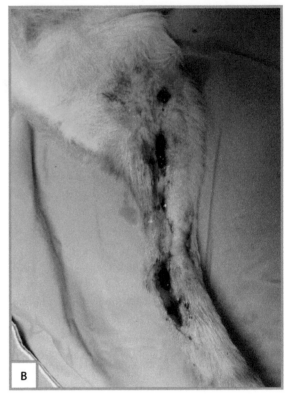

Figure 1.2 Photographs of an open, grade IIIB, highly comminuted, fracture of the diaphysis and distal metaphysis of the distal tibia. (A) preoperative image. Bone loss is present and the fracture included the distal articular surface. Although this limb was salvaged (B) postoperative image, the tibial tarsal joint was arthrodesed and lameness was always present.

doses; preferably within three hours of injury. If there is much contamination, an aminoglycoside should be added. Grade III open fractures should always be treated with a first generation cephalosporin and an aminoglycoside. In the case of contamination from heavy soil or fecal matter (for example, after farm injuries), metronidazole or clindamycin should also be administered for anaerobic coverage. The antibiotics should be administered for a maximum of 72 hours. Some surgeons discontinue antibiotics sooner; at the time of first debridement or soft tissue closure. A longer course of antibiotic therapy is not indicated and encourages antibiotic resistance. Infection rates have been reported as 2.3 percent for grade I and II fractures versus 17.6 percent for grade III.[12]

Fracture location and configuration have a large impact on overall assessment and implant choice. The bone involved gives rise to considerations of both mechanics and biology. For example, surgical fixation of the pelvis has the advantage of a good

blood supply and shorter bone levers acting on the fractures. Muscles of the pelvis often act to splint fractures. However, attention to impingement of the pelvic canal due to displacement, malunion, or large callus formation must still be considered. Femoral fractures have a good blood supply, but are subjected to large forces. The humerus has large and complex forces acting on it including bending and torsion. Fixation techniques that counter all fracture forces must be chosen to yield the best prognosis. The tibia has primarily axial loads and several basic repair implant devices are available. However, the distal tibia is the primary site for non-unions in humans and can be problematic in animals as well. Blood supply to the distal radius can be scant in small breed dogs which commonly results in delayed or non-unions.[5] The metaphyseal region of many bones is rich in well-vascularized cancellous bone and has good healing potential which often allows for less rigid fixation methods. Salter fractures occur in the metaphyseal region of bones and have the advantage of a rich blood supply. By definition, Salter fractures occur in young animals associated with mechanically stable fracture configurations. In such cases, simple pin fixation can be successful, but must be applied to allow continued bone growth at the physes.

The amount of energy imparted to a fracture is an important consideration during assessment. The more energy imparted to the fracture, the larger amount of bone and soft tissue compromised. Gunshot wounds are good examples of this effect.[13] A 0.22 long rifle round often has a 2.6 g lead slug and a muzzle velocity of 370 m/s with an energy of 141 J. By comparison, a 0.223 caliber (5.56 × 45 mm) round has a 2 g bullet, but a muzzle velocity of 1,140 m/s and an energy of 1.524 J. For a comparable size of slug, the second round has over ten times the energy of the first. In low velocity gunshot wounds, the fracture is treated essentially as a closed fracture.[12] In contrast, high velocity gunshot wounds must be treated as grade III open fractures. These carry a much greater risk of infection, non-union, and soft tissue damage. Nerve damage is frequent. The wound must be debrided and copiously lavaged. The wound is often left open.

Motor vehicle accidents impart considerable energy to bone and soft tissues depending on the velocity of the collision, size of patient, manner of impact, and whether the patient was run over by the vehicle. The degree of fracture comminution is an indicator of impact energy. Bone deformation is load-rate dependent; it bends differently based on the rate it is loaded. Bone is both viscoelastic and viscoplastic. If bone is loaded quickly, it is stiffer and will absorb more energy. When bone does fail, the energy is imparted throughout the loaded and deformed bone, resulting in more comminution. Bone loaded slowly tends to have more simple fracture characteristics and implies lower total energy imparted to the location. Also, the transfer of more energy from a high velocity fracture will result in more comminution. For these reasons, a highly comminuted fracture suggests a higher energy fracture and more trauma to both bone and soft tissue. Clinical consequences are less viable soft tissues which are more susceptible to infection and have a slower vascular recovery. There is subsequently retarded fracture healing. Skin and other soft tissues may die and need debridement. A higher energy fracture can be anticipated to require more time to heal, be more likely to require bone grafting either at the time of fixation or later during healing, and have a greater propensity for infection.

The skin of dogs and cats is relatively mobile so motor vehicle trauma can result in devitalized skin areas from tire pressure. Skin can therefore be devitalized with minimal energy absorption by the patient itself. Large areas of traumatized skin may subsequently die, requiring plastic procedures to close the defect. A patient completely run over by a vehicle often has considerable soft tissue injury. Vital structures inclusive within the urinary and gastrointestinal tracts may be injured and further compromise healing of fractures. A pelvic fracture with multiple fracture sites and comminution indicates an especially high-energy transfer.

The extent of soft tissue injury is often directly related to the energy of the injury; external forces great enough to fracture bone must first traverse through soft tissue. In contrast, fractures caused by a knife or axe (which are rare), may not have substantial associated soft tissue damage.

Fracture Classification

A fracture should be described using precise terminology and in a given sequence of descriptors. This allows accurate communication between clinicians and accurate medical records accuracy. The order of terms are:

1. Whether the fracture is open or closed.
2. The fracture configuration.
3. Location of the fracture within the bone.
4. The specific bone fractured.
5. Displacement and over-riding presence.

A fracture is first described as open or closed and when open, its degree. The configuration of the fracture is then described; transverse, oblique, or comminuted. Transverse fractures are those perpendicular to the long axis of the bone, whereas other fractures would be oblique. Oblique fractures should be classified as short or long. An oblique fracture is defined as long when the length of obliquity is twice the diameter of the bone, and short when the obliquity is less than that. Differentiating between long and short oblique fractures significantly impacts on the choice of implant. All oblique fractures are subjected to shear forces during healing, and since most long-bone force is axial, the longer the obliquity, the greater the shear force.

Fracture location in a specific bone refers primarily to its metaphyseal or diaphyseal location. If metaphyseal, then the proximal or distal location should be noted.

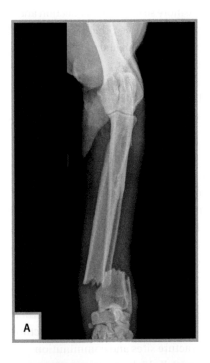

A

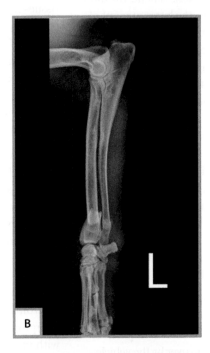

B

Figure 1.3 Radiographs of a closed, transverse fracture of the distal quarter of the diphysis of the radius, displaced laterally and over-riding 10 mm (A) preoperative: cranial/caudal view; (B) preoperative: lateral view.

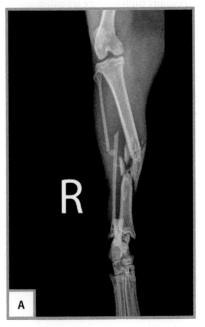

A

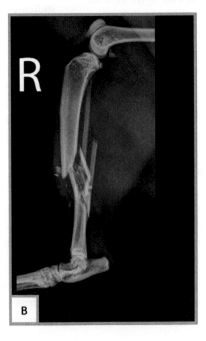

B

Figure 1.4 Radiographs of a grade II open, highly comminuted fracture of the mid diaphysis of the tibia, displaced laterally and over-riding 15 mm. (A) preoperative: cranial/caudal view; (B) preoperative: lateral view.

If the location is diaphyseal, then approximately which segment of the diaphysis (proximal quarter, mid-diaphyseal, or distal quarter) should also be noted.

The specific bone(s) fractured should then be noted. Logically, the bone in question would be noted first; however, the accepted custom is to first list the qualifiers above prior to identifying the specific bone. The next descriptor is displacement and over-riding (in millimeters) of the fracture. Always, the position of the distal fragment dictates the direction of displacement in orthogonal directions. These would be either cranial or caudal, then medial or lateral (compare Figures 1.3–1.6).

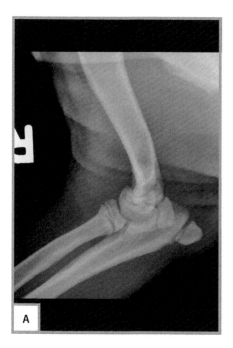

A

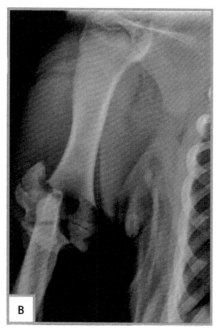

B

Figure 1.5 Radiographs of a closed, Salter IV fracture of the distal humeral condyle. The capitulum is displaced laterally and over-riding 5 mm. (A) preoperative: cranial/caudal view; (B) preoperative: lateral view.

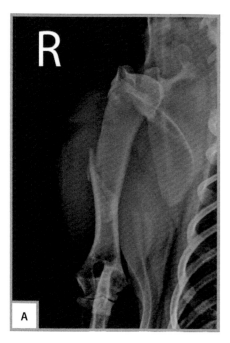

A

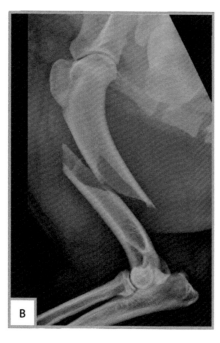

B

Figure 1.6 Radiographs of a closed, long oblique fracture of the diaphysis of the humerus, displaced laterally and over-riding 2 cm. (A) preoperative: cranial/caudal view; (B) preoperative: lateral view.

Forces Acting on Bone and the Fracture

Normal bone is subjected to continual loads which are supported by means of forces. Changes to normal loads have to be countered by forces with equal and opposite force. These forces include tension (axial force), compression (axial force), shear, bending, and flexure, (torsion). It may be helpful to think of bone as a wall made up of bricks and mortar (see schematics shown in Figures 1.7–1.10). The bricks represent the mineral component of bone and the mortar represents collagen. An axial load is the load produced by pushing on the ends of long bones. The direction of gravity as well as the structure of the skeletal system and pull of muscles results in long bones being subjected to loads orientated along the long axial, hence, these are referred to as axial loads. One can liken this to a force pushing down on the wall (Figure 1.7).

Compression loads are typically much larger than other loads. As such, bone is able to counter relatively large axial force. Fixation constructs must be equally stout in providing optimal strength and stiffness to counter these forces to enable bone healing.

Tension or tensile forces are those that distract a bone. They separate the joint surfaces without rupture, for example, as facilitated by the attachment of muscles by tendons. Using the wall analogy again, tensile forces are those that would lift a brick off the wall. Whilst bone can sustain large compressive forces, far less force is required to pull apart a section of bone (Figure 1.8).

Shear forces are those exerting opposite directional, but unaligned, forces on a structure. If these forces were directly opposite in alignment, they would be compressive. Since they are not aligned, these forces tend to cause a shifting or sliding of one part of a structure against another part of the same structure. Shear forces can disrupt bone healing[14] and can be thought of, in the context of the brick wall analogy, as pushing on one section of the brick and mortar wall and having one group of bricks slide along another group, as shown in Figure 1.9.

Bending is the result of a combination of both compressive and tensile forces. As a cylindrical beam is bent, for example, tensile forces act on one side of the beam and compressive forces on the opposite side. In the center, there will be no compressive or tensile forces. This is called the neutral plane. There will be various directions and magnitudes of compressive and tensile forces throughout the structure due to bending, resulting

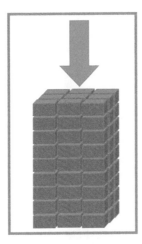

Figure 1.7 Schematic illustrating analogy of bone as a brick wall and the effects of forces acting on it. The bricks represent the mineral component and the mortar, the collagen. Such a structure is very strong under axial loads due to compression forces (indicated by the direction of the blue arrow).

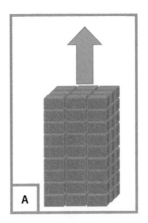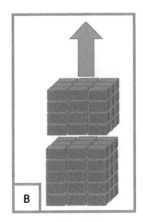

Figure 1.8 Schematic illustrating how traction is a tensile force on bone (blue arrow indicates force direction) (A). Fractures due to tension forces are usually simple and transverse (B).

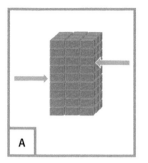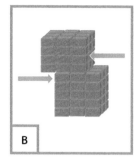

A   B

Figure 1.9 Schematic illustrating that shear forces are opposite in direction but occur in the same plane (blue arrows indicate force directions) (A). Bone is relatively weak with regard to its ability to withstand the stress imposed by shear forces (B).

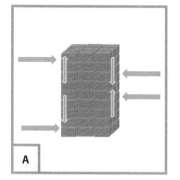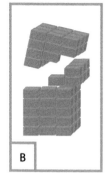

A   B

Figure 1.10 Schematic illustrating four point bending (A). Bending is a combination of forces which results in compression on one side of the structure and tension on the other. In the center there is neither compression nor tension and this is the neutral plane. However, because there are varying degrees and direction of forces in the bending structure, shear forces develop within. Since the bone is weakest in tension, the fracture starts on the tension side, but generally does not progress transversely. Due to the internal shear forces, comminution of the fracture is likely and fragments often develop (B).

in shear stresses between adjacent areas. Bone is best able to accommodate compressive forces, less able to accommodate tensile forces, and quite poor at accommodating shear forces. Accordingly, in fractures subjected to bending, a partially transverse fracture in the area of bone subjected to tension is accompanied by obliquity or fragmentation from shear forces in the area of bone subjected to compression (Figure 1.10). Using the wall analogy again, pushing at the top of the wall would result in the mortar separating on the side of the wall that was being pushed. If ever asked to knock down a wall, the easiest method would be by using a bending force.

Finally, torsional forces are those that twist bone. This force also results in compressive and tensile forces, but over the length of the bone. Bone fracture therefore occurs over a longer bone length and often results in long oblique or spiral oblique fractures.

Mechanics of Orthopedic Devices

Knowledge of some basic material mechanics is useful in understanding how best to leverage mechanics in the choice of a device for fracture repair.[15] The properties of a device are dictated by the material composition and its shape. There are two main materials used in orthopedic devices: 316 L (Low carbon) stainless steel and grade 5 titanium. 316 L stainless steel is the most common material used; it is biologically compatible, strong with some flexibility, tolerant to contouring and inexpensive. Grade 5 titanium is an alloy with 6 percent aluminum and 4 percent vanadium which is abbreviated Ti-Al6-V4. Titanium is lighter per unit volume than 316 L stainless steel, and stronger per unit weight. Titanium is also more elastic. If identical plates were made from these two materials, they would have similar strengths but the plate made from 316 L stainless steel would be heavier, and the Ti-Al6-V4 plate would have greater elasticity.

AMI is the property of a two-dimensional plane shape that characterizes the expected deflection of that shape when loaded. A surgeon can use these criteria to judge how an implant will perform and to help compare the relative performance of different sizes of three-dimensional implants. All shapes have an AMI and a shape can have loads applied in different directions. However, rods (pins, connecting rods, screws) or bars (plates) commonly represent orthopedic devices. The AMI of rods and rectangular beams are provided in Figures 1.11 and 1.12.

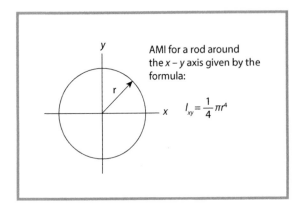

Figure 1.11 Schematic illustrating the AMI of a rod. The cross-sectional area is shown and represents an external fixator pin or minor (inner) diameter of a screw. If the shape is elongated and bent around the x and y axes, then the relationship of the shape to its stiffness is given by the formula $I_{xy} = \frac{1}{4}\pi r^4$. Note that stiffness is related to the radius to the fourth power; if the diameter of a rod or screw is doubled, then the stiffness increases by a factor of 16.

In Figure 1.11, the lines x and y represent two orthogonal axes, around which the elongated shape can be bent. The radius of the circle affects the AMI to the fourth power. Relating this to a three-dimensional rod, a doubling of the diameter of a rod or pin will increase the AMI by 16 times. With most materials, this relates to a 16-fold increase in strength and stiffness. Since the diameter of rods have such a profound influence on AMI, if greater strength and stiffness is desired then even small increases in the diameter of a pin or screw will often have a profound effect. Conversely, as implants become smaller, the AMI is affected negatively to the fourth power. Consider how this is applied clinically. Presume a 20 kg dog has a 10 mm diameter tibia and a 40 kg dog has a 20 mm diameter tibia. If an external fixator pin is chosen to be 20 percent of the diameter of the bone, selected pins would be 2.0 mm and 4.0 mm in diameter, respectively. But the stiffness of the 4.0 mm pin is 16 times that of the 2.0 mm pin, while the larger dog is only twice as heavy. The surgeon can choose to use comparatively larger pins, or a more robust construct with more pins for the smaller dog.

In the case of the rectangle as shown in Figure 1.12, increasing the height of the rectangle will increase the AMI to the third power, yet bending around the

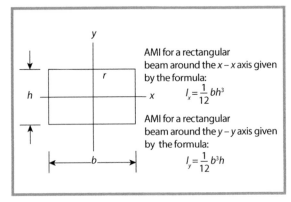

Figure 1.12 Schematic illustrating the AMI of a rectangular beam. The cross-sectional area is shown and represents a bone plate. If the shape is elongated and bent around the x axis then the relationship of the shape to its stiffness is given by the formula $I_x = \frac{1}{12}bh^3$. Note that stiffness is related to the plate's thickness (h) to the third power. If the shape is elongated and bent around the y axis then the relationship of the shape to its stiffness is given by the formula $I_y = \frac{1}{12}b^3h$. There is a linear relationship between the plate's width (b) and stiffness. If the thickness of the plate is doubled, then the stiffness increases by a factor of 8; if the width is doubled then the stiffness increases by a factor of 2.

x-axis while increasing the width is simply a linear relationship. This relates to clinical bone plating, in that increasing the thickness of a plate will have a profoundly larger influence on the strength and stiffness of the plate compared to increasing its width. Using a larger and thicker plate would yield a much greater influence on strength and stiffness than using two plates, side by side, in the same plane.

The relative influences of shape on AMI can be used to estimate the effects of dimensions from complex shapes, such as two plates in orthogonal planes. An example would be one plate on the cranial aspect, together with one plate on the medial side of a radius. The effects of these two orthogonal plates would have a much greater influence than two plates lying side by side. This is known as the 'I' beam effect, where plates at orthogonal planes greatly enhance strength and stiffness without large increases in weight.

Other mechanical principles that can be employed to estimate or compare different orthopedic devices or constructs are beam mechanics.

Figure 1.13 depicts a beam fixed to a supportive structure. The beam can be thought of as an external fixator pin or screw in a locking plate. The equation $x(mm) = \dfrac{64\,PL^3}{3\pi d^4}$ gives the amount of deflection at the end of the beam when a force is applied. The distance from the supportive structure at which the load is applied will increase the amount of deflection to the third power. Therefore, if a single half-pin in an external fixator or a single screw in a locking plate is used, doubling the distance from the connecting rod (or plate to bone) will allow eight times more deflection with a load applied to that screw or pin. All efforts should be made to keep that distance short for both types of fixation construct.

Even well-contoured plates will be subjected to bending forces and those forces will increase exponentially as the plate moves farther from the center of the bone or the neutral axis. For this reason adding an IM pin can greatly increase the stiffness and strength of the fixation construct and will decrease stresses on the plate. This is the principle of 'plate-rod constructs'.

A list of basic orthopedic devices, a list of rules, explanation of these rules, advisement for implementation and basic application techniques now follows. This is just a foundation for understanding. This text is not meant to be a definitive orthopedic fracture repair text, but rather, a reference for examples of basic fractures and successful repairs. Assuredly, not all devices are listed. Neither are all different types of a specific device described. A surgeon should acquire all relevant information and training on the specifics of each orthopedic device and the nuances of indications and application for use.

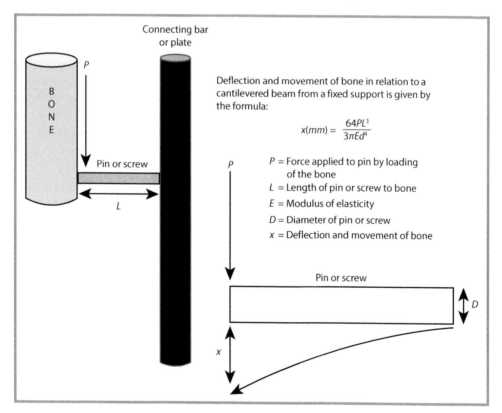

Figure 1.13 Schematic illustrating the relationship between a single beam in cantilever bending and the distance to the force. An external fixator pin or a screw in a locking plate system is shown. As the distance from the supporting column (connecting bar or plate) increases, the amount of deflection and movement of the bone, for a given force and diameter of screw or pin is given by the formula $x(mm) = \dfrac{64PL^3}{3\pi Ed^4}$. Note that increasing the inner diameter of the screw or fixator pin will decrease the amount of deflection to the fourth power.

Cerclage Wire

Rules for Using Cerclage Wire

1. Fractures must be long oblique; obliquity–twice the diameter of the bone.
2. Cerclage is not to be the sole means of repair.
3. As large as practical cerclage wire should be used. 1.0–1.2 mm (18–20 guage) in dogs and 0.64–0.81 mm (20–22 gauge) in small (toy) dog breeds and cats.
4. Two or more circumferential cerclage wires must be used; placed 8–10 mm apart.
5. Cerclage should be no closer than 5 mm from the fracture ends.
6. Wire must reside directly on the bone and confirmed to be tight.

The function of a cerclage wire is to encircle sections of bone and compress them as shown in Figure 1.14.[16] The mechanical principle is similar to a wooden barrel (the components of a barrel are the staves, hoops, and stave joints). Staves form a cylinder and steel hoops actively press the staves together. In a barrel, if the hoop is not taut and pressing the staves together, or if a stave joint fails, then the integrity of the barrel is lost. The wooden staves are like segments of bone, stave joints are like fracture lines, and the hoop is analogous to the cerclage wire.

Mechanically, a segment of bone repaired with cerclage wire relies upon these three components functioning together; bone fragments reconstructed into the cylinder, stable fracture lines, and tight cerclage. If any of these requirements is not met or fails, then the construct becomes unstable. Loose cerclage wire and unstable bone fragments are a common cause of non-unions.

The bone fragments must be included in a 'reconstructible' repair. If there are missing segments of bone (of even modest size), then the integrity of the cylinder will be lost and the cerclage wire cannot compress the fracture lines. Unlike a barrel, fracture lines are typically not always perpendicular to the cerclage wire. Compression provided by cerclage wire that is not perpendicular to a fracture line will cause shear forces between the fracture fragments. Motion due to the imposed shear forces must be countered by friction at the interfragmentary fracture line. The farther from perpendicular, the greater the required friction to prevent fracture collapse. Typically, if the fracture line is a short oblique (see Fracture Classification section) then cerclage wire will be far from perpendicular to the fracture lines and failure due to shear forces will occur. The longer the obliquity, the lesser the shear forces and the more stable the fracture line.

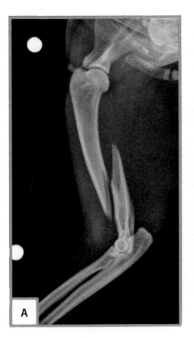
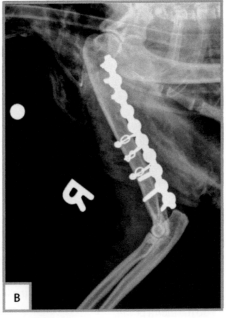

Figure 1.14 Radiographs of a long oblique fracture of the humerus ((A) preoperative: lateral view) repaired using cerclage wires supported by a locking plate ((B) postoperative: lateral view). Note that the repair uses more than one (1.2 mm) wire; the cerclage wire is loop cerclage wire; the first wire is no closer than 5 mm from the fracture end and subsequent wires are 1 cm apart. The cerclage wire is also tight on the bone.

The fracture can also become unstable if the fragments are able to pivot on a cerclage wire. Use of single cerclage wires can allow pivoting that leads to instability. More than one cerclage wire must be used. Also, even if more than one cerclage wire is placed, bending forces can dislodge a bone fragment leading to wire loosening. For this reason cerclage wire should not be used as a sole method of fracture fixation.

Cerclage wire must not enter a fracture line; this will distract the fracture. Cerclage wire must be placed some distance from the end of a fracture line and a somewhat arbitrary but common rule is to place cerclage wire no closer than 5 mm to the fracture end.

Cerclage wire actively compresses bone across fracture lines. In order for this to occur, the cerclage must be made of the proper material, consist of the proper size, and be applied correctly. 316 L (not spring-hardened) stainless steel with an appropriate modulus of elasticity is commonly used. Hardening 316 stainless steel, as is the process for pins and Kirschner wire, increases the stiffness and decreases the elasticity. The larger the size of the wire, the greater the elasticity before yield. The largest size that retains clinical manageability should therefore be used. Typically, this is no smaller than 0.8 mm (20 gauge). In large dogs, 1 mm (18 gauge) and 1.2 mm (16 gauge) wire are the most appropriate.

Cerclage wire is applied perpendicular to the long axis of the bone and not in an area of conical shape, as the wire is more apt to slip, or loosen. A full configuration of cerclage wire is preferred although hemi-cerclage, wire suture, and other configurations of cerclage wire have been described. Cerclage configurations, other than full are more apt to loosen. Movement of loose cerclage wire has the potential to sever blood supply to the periosteum and contribute to non-union.

Methods for tightening cerclage wire, including loop, double loop, and twisting,[17, 18] have been studied. The cerclage wire should be positioned in contact with the bone and with minimal inclusive soft tissue (best positioned with a wire passer).

Regardless of the method of tensioning and securing the wire it should be secured so as to be as tight as possible. Breaking wires during application can occur; broken wires are simply replaced. When cerclage wire is secured by twisting, the twisted ends should *not* be bent over after twisting, as this loosens the wire. However, bending wire close to bone remains a common surgical practice with some surgeons advocating the bending of the wire in the same motion as that completed in the last twist to maintain the tightness of the wire. The wire should be cut with 2–3 twists remaining.

Cerclage wires cause interfragmentary compression and when applied correctly, can prevent shearing when axial forces are applied to the bone. Given the correct fracture configuration, cerclage wires can aid in resisting bending forces on a fracture.

Cerclage wire is best suited for long oblique fractures of the tibia, femur, and humerus. It should be avoided when dealing with grade III open fractures, as well as comminuted fractures. Cerclage wire must be applied correctly to avoid iatrogenic non-unions.

Intramedullary Pins

Rules for Intramedullary (IM) Pins

1. Pins should be 50–75 percent of the diameter of the medullary cavity in the area of the fracture.[19]
2. Pins should be placed normograde when possible.[20]
3. Pins should be seated in the trans- (far) epiphysis.
4. Any fixation construct should counter torsional stress, or ancillary devices should be employed.
5. If IM pins are used in conjunction with plates (plate-rod configuration), the size of the pin should be 30–50 percent the diameter of the medullary cavity.

Non-locking IM pins have long been used in fracture fixation. The medullary cavity is in the center of the bone, running through the longitudinal axis. Because of this, IM pins are very strong in opposing loads along their long axis. IM pins are also in the neutral plane in bending. As such, IM pins are in a mechanically favorable location to counter bending-loads. These pins can be comparatively large and therefore very stiff and strong. Another factor to consider is that IM pins are very economical.

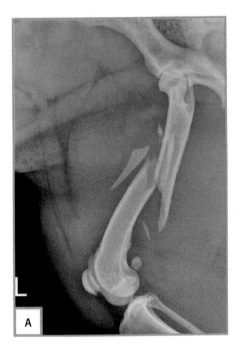

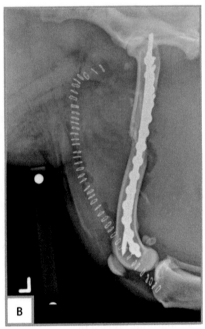

Figure 1.15 Radiographs of an IM pin used to support plating of a comminuted femoral fracture in a plate/rod construct. The pin was placed normograde and is approximately half the diameter of the medullary cavity at mid-diaphysis. (A) preoperative: lateral view; (B) postoperative: lateral view.

IM pins do not, however, counter torsional forces. Even if more than one IM pin is used (stack pinning), the effect on torsional stiffness is minimal unless the medullary cavity is completely filled, which may result in IM blood flow being compromised.[21] For this reason IM pins are best used with other fixation devices (Figure 1.15).

In comparison with smooth IM pins, interlocking nails are an improved device, as transfer members (screws or bolts), provide increased stiffness especially against torsional forces (Figure 1.16).[22–24]

IM pins are best placed normograde; from the ends of the bone and not initially introduced from the fracture site. Pins placed from the fracture line and driven in the opposite direction (retrograde) to seat in the opposite epiphyses may result in inappropriate positioning as the pin exits the bone. A common example of this is placement of an IM pin in the femur. If placed retrograde, the pin tends to exit the femur in close proximity to the sciatic nerve. Further, retrograde-imposed medial diversion of the pin renders it more difficult to cut, leaving excess pin length to cause soft tissue trauma. Excessive reaming of the medullary canal should be avoided with IM pins or interlocking nails.[19, 25]

The intertrochanteric fossa is the location for femoral normograde pin placement. In the humerus, pins can be placed distally from the medial epicondyle, or proximally at the greater tubercle. Normograded ulnar pins are introduced at the olecranon. Pins are introduced into the tibia from a location half-way between the tibial tuberosity and the medial collateral ligament on the tibial plateau. Pins are rarely placed into the radius and often result in complications.

IM pins are preferably placed with a low-speed (high-torque) drill. Placing pins using a hand chuck is acceptable, but greater 'wobble' is likely. First the fracture is reduced, then the pin is placed until the tip of the pin is seated in the far epiphysis. It is best to place the pin along a cortex; placing the pin in the center of the medullary canal provides less stability. The pin is cut as close as possible to the bone entry site.

Dynamic Compression Plates[26]

Rules for Dynamic Compression Plating

1. Appropriate plate size is generally dictated by the size of the screw allowed. The major diameter of the screw (outside diameter) should

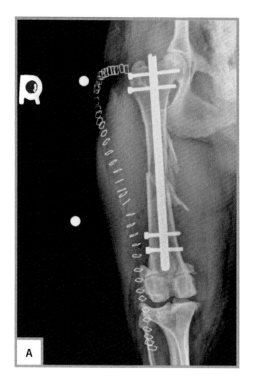

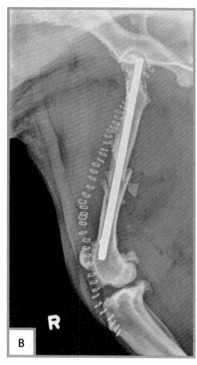

Figure 1.16 Radiographs of a locking IM nail used with bolts. The nail is in the neutral plane in the center of the bone. The bolts prevent collapse of the fracture and in theory prevent rotational movement from torsional forces. (A) postoperative: cranial/caudal view; (B) postoperative: cranial/caudal view.

approach, but be no greater than 20 percent of the diameter of the bone being plated.

2. Screws should engage at least six cortices on either side of a fracture.
3. Screws should engage both cis- (near) and trans- (far) cortices.
4. The fracture should be reduced, so that there is cortical contact, especially on the trans-cortex.
5. The plate should be contoured so that it lies directly on the bone.
6. Screws should be placed in 'load position'; away from the fracture line in the dynamic compression hole.

Dynamic compression plates (DCPs) are applied so that the screws in the plate compress the fracture fragments, and weight-bearing allows load sharing and dynamic compression across fracture lines during healing. Plates provide support in all degrees of freedom including bending, torsion and shear. Bone is best suited to counter forces due to axial loads and primary bone healing can be achieved with rigid fixation as fracture segment compression is achieved with DCPs. However, for the plate to effectively impose dynamic compression, the fracture segments must be opposed; especially on the trans-cortex. If there is a fracture gap on the trans-cortex, then the fracture may collapse or alternatively the plate may deform elastically, causing high cyclic-strain in these fracture gaps. The application of a plate in dynamic compression usually requires open reduction for proper fracture reduction prior to plate application. This involves soft tissues invasion with compromise of the biological environment. DCPs need not always be used in compression, but can be applied as buttress devices or as a load-sharing device without eliciting dynamic compression.[27]

DCPs are the best choice for transverse, closed, minimally-to-non-comminuted fractures that can be accurately reduced. A classic example is a transverse or very short oblique fracture of the radius, femur, or tibia as seen in Figure 1.17.

DCPs can be applied using a variety of mechanical methods. Buttress fashion is where a plate is applied to counter all loads in order that a fracture does not assume any weight-bearing load until it is bridged. Alternatively, a fracture can be reduced and supported by a plate but the fracture and plate share the load of weight-bearing, although load is not dynamically imparted to the fracture. Using a

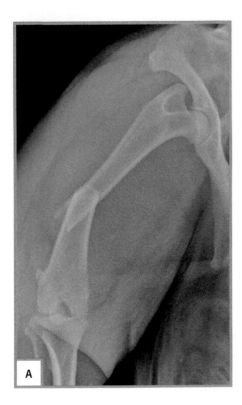

A

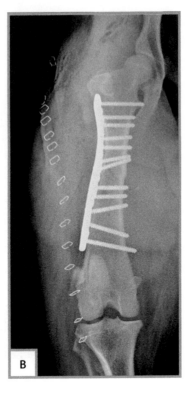

B

Figure 1.17 Radiographs of a DCP used to stabilize a short oblique femoral fracture ((A) preoperative: lateral view). Two screws are placed in lag fashion across the fracture. Properly applied, a DCP will allow forces to compress the fracture lines during normal ambulation ((B) postoperative: cranial/caudal view).

DCP allows for dynamic compression; the plate is positioned such that the bone assumes the majority of the axial load during weight-bearing.

When applying a plate in dynamic compression, the bone is first exposed. The fracture is reduced and then an appropriate plate is selected that will allow at least six cortices of screw purchase on each side of the fracture line. The plate is contoured so that it lies as congruently against the bone as possible. Inappropriate contouring of plates can produce asymmetric compression, where the cis-cortex is compressed more than the trans-cortex. It is mechanically advantageous to have greater compression at the trans-cortex. It is possible by bending the plate in order that it lies slightly elevated from the bone at the fracture area to allow a bending moment on the bone ends and compression of the trans-cortices. This is achieved because when the screws are inserted into such a plate, it is elastically pulled to the bone. The plate should be raised about 1 mm for a 3.5 mm plate and 2 mm for a 4.5 mm plate. When placing a plate in compression, screws closer to the fracture line are placed first. The first hole is drilled on one side of the fracture. The depth of the screw hole is measured, and 2 mm is added to this measurement for screw selection. More length should be added to self-tapping screws since the flutes remove bone/screw purchase. Less screw length is used if the plate is significantly pre-bent or another bone or structure is immediately on the other side of the trans-cortex (for example, fibula on the distant side of the tibia, or ulna on the distant side of the radius). The hole is tapped if non-self-tapping screws are used. If the bone is particularly dense, a tap is better able to create threads and remove bone debris than a self-tapping screw. If self-tapping screws are used, then they should have three cutting flutes. The screw is fully inserted, then counter-rotated one revolution. The plate is pushed toward the fracture and a loading drill guide is used for positioning the screw in compression. Again, the hole is measured, tapped, and the screw is inserted. After all screws are placed, they are tightened alternately on either side of the fracture line and the degree of compression, especially at the trans-cortex, is assessed. Additional screws are placed next to the first and in compression if more compression is needed. Each screw applied in load fashion can move or track the bone 0.8 mm for a 2.7 mm plate and 1.0 mm for a 3.5 mm plate. However, no more than two screws should be placed in load fashion on either side of the fracture. In addition, this amount of compression may be too much if the fracture is already reduced and compressed. If the fracture lines are already compressed, additional screws are not placed in load. Additional screws are placed neutrally but still with the screw in the hole and away from the fracture.

Locking Plates

Rules for Applying Locking Plates

1. Appropriate plate size is generally dictated by the size of the screw allowed; the major diameter of the screw should approach, but be no greater than 20 percent of the diameter of the bone being plated.
2. Three, or preferably four, screws should engage bone on either side of the fracture.[28]
3. Unicortical screws can be used.
4. The plate must not lie directly on the bone, but should be as close as possible.
5. Ancillary devices such as IM pins or second plates should be considered.[29]

The mechanics of locking plates is somewhat different than dynamic compression plating.[24, 28, 30–33] The screws are angle stable and should not pivot in the screw hole.[34] It is helpful to think of the plate as an external fixator under the skin. The screws follow the principles of beam mechanics described above. Also, the screws do not pull the plate to the bone, but rather multiple screws hold the bone in a fixed position relative to the plate. In order for the plate to be pulled off the bone, the screw must slice through the bone rather than being stripped out of the bone as occurs with DCP plate screws. Locking screws hold better in soft bone. In addition, if a screw in DCP application engages only one cortex, load causes that screw to pivot in the screw hole of that single cortex. Damage of the bone/screw interface is likely. If the screw is angle-stable and the interface between the screw and plate is rigid (as occurs with interlocking mechanics), then the screw will tend not to pivot and damage to the bone/screw interface is less likely. For this reason, unicortical screws are used in locking plates with greater utility than in standard DCP plates.

Locking plates counter all forces (axial, bending, torsion, shear and tension) on fractured bone.

The angle stability of locking screws does increase the strain at the screw/plate interface. This can result in screw breakage or dislodging of the screw from the plate. These forces can be minimized by increasing the number of screws in the construct.

Locking plates are always used as buttress devices. They never result in dynamic compression. In addition, locking plates may elastically bend and recoil during loading. This may encourage healing, as some motion is occurring at the fracture site. If, however, this motion exceeds the upper limit of strain tolerated by the healing bone, osteosynthesis can be adversely affected.

Locking plates do not need absolute contouring to bone, and since they are buttress devices, absolute anatomic reduction of the fracture is not required. For these reasons, locking plates are used in highly comminuted fractures or with minimally invasive fracture fixation techniques such as Minimally Invasive Plate Osteosynthesis (MIPO) (Figure 1.18).[35–37] Such plates are commonly used on comminuted femoral fractures, humeral fractures, soft and/or juvenile bone, and thin bones such as the scapula or ilium.

External Fixators[8]

Rules for Applying External Fixators

1. The appropriate external fixator (EF) type is generally dictated by the size of the fixation pin allowed; the major diameter of the fixation pin should approach, but be no greater than 20 percent of the diameter of the bone being plated.
2. Full pins (penetrating both the cis- and trans-cortex) should be used when possible. Alternatively, double connecting rods with half-pins (Type Ib configuration) fixators can be used.
3. Three pins should engage bone on each side of the fracture.

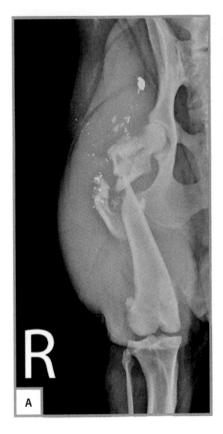

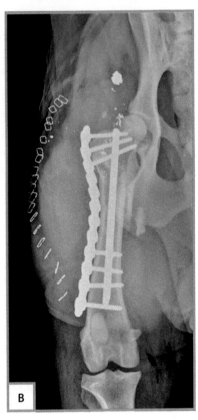

Figure 1.18 Radiographs of a locking plate with angle-stable screws used to stabilize a grade II, open, highly comminuted fracture of the proximal femur ((A) preoperative: cranial/caudal view) using a plate/rod construct ((B) postoperative: cranial/caudal view). Angle-stable screws are better able to hold softer metaphyseal bone.

4. Positive profile pins should be used and pilot holes for transfixation pins should be pre-drilled.
5. Pins should be placed perpendicular to the long axis of bone when possible.
6. Pins should be placed near the ends of the bone, as well as close to the fracture.
7. Large connecting rods should be used.
8. Clamps should be placed close to, but not touching, the skin.

External fixators are buttress devices where weight-bearing load is transmitted from the limb, to fixation pins, to the connecting column, then back to the bone on the other side of the fracture.[38] In contrast to locking plates, fixators are external to the skin. This presents two major issues. First, EF transfixation pins penetrate skin and therefore allow healing bone access to external bacterial contamination. Infection can lead to skin irritation around the entry site of the pin and bone resorption along the pin tract. The second issue relates to the distance of the transfixation pin from the fractured bone to the connecting rod. The diameter, and therefore strength and stiffness of the transfixation pin is limited to a diameter that is approximately 20 percent of the diameter of the bone. Transfixation pins are also made of a material which has greater stiffness than regular IM pins though both are typically 316L stainless steel. The distance from the connecting column to the bone is the limiting factor in the support provided by the fixator (see Figure 1.13). Remember that the amount of deflection of a beam is related to its length to the third power. Therefore, even small increases in the length from bone to connecting column result in a geometric decrease in stiffness of the construct. Even though the connecting columns are placed close to skin, this distance can be quite large in upper limb bones such as the femur and humerus. Compensation for this weakness is substitution of half-pins with full pins; pins that pass completely through the limb and attach on either side of the limb to connecting rods (such constructs are limited to below the elbow and below the knee). This Type II construct dramatically increases the strength and stiffness of the fixator.[38, 39] Other options are to incorporate

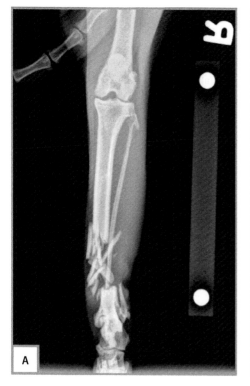

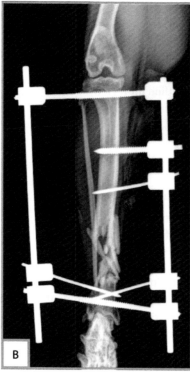

Figure 1.19 Radiographs of a closed, highly comminuted fracture of the distal fourth of the tibia ((A) preoperative: cranial/caudal view) stabilized using a bilateral, Type II external fixator ((B) postoperative: lateral view) Full pins provide greater stiffness compared to half-pins and three pins engage both the proximal and distal segments. Pins are placed at the bone ends and as close to the fracture as possible.

IM pins; which, again, act to support the cantilever bending of the half-pins.

Fixators, therefore, have greatest efficacy when the length of the transfixation pin is relatively short and when full pins or other supportive techniques can be employed. They have, therefore, most utility in the distal limb; specifically the tibia and radius/ulna (Figure 1.19).

The bone/pin interface can be easily compromised by both infection and poor mechanical stability. Infection causes bone reabsorption and mechanical instability results in increased bone/pin interface strain and damage to this interface. For this reason, integrity of the bone/pin interface should be retained as much as possible. This is achieved using a combination of application principles including threaded pins, pre-drilling the pin holes, using three or more pins per bone segment, and placing transfixation pins perpendicular to the long axis of the bone to counter shear forces.

An external fixator should be placed using a sequence of standard procedures. First, a pin is placed in one epiphysis close to the joint, then a further pin is placed in the opposite epiphysis of the same fractured long bone. Connecting bars are fastened to the transfixation pins and the fracture is aligned. Typically, fracture alignment is performed in this sequence: axial, or translational alignment, then medial-to-lateral bending, then torsional alignment, followed by cranial-to-caudal bending. Thereafter, additional transfixation pins are applied, with at least three per bone segment. More support structures may be added for additional strength.

An additional advantage of external fixators is that the stiffness of the fixator can be changed during healing by removing fixation pins, or preferably by axial dynamization, where the axial stiffness is reduced without effecting bending or torsional stiffness.[40]

There are many other notable fixation devices that are used in fracture repair, notably ring fixators and interlocking nails. Each specific device has preferred application methods, based on the recommendations of the designer, which should be adhered to.

Evaluation of Postoperative Radiographs

Radiographs must be evaluated critically to anticipate potential complications and improve techniques. A standard method for reviewing the images is to consider in turn the four 'A's: Alignment, Apposition, Apparatus, and Activity.

Alignment

Alignment is the overall 'straightening up' of the fractured bone. Fractures are not always anatomically reduced; surgical exposure to accomplish alignment may impair the biological environment for fracture healing. However, bones must be aligned so that function can be restored and the potential for healing optimized. Alignment is evaluated with respect to axial, cranial-to-caudal bending, medial-to-lateral bending, and rotation. Axial alignment is particularly important. This is the position of the proximal and distal epiphyses of the bone in relation to the central axis of the bone. Failure to re-establish the correct axial alignment will result in improper loading of the limb, lameness, and dysfunction.

In the forelimb there are the shoulder, elbow, and carpal joints. In the caudal limb there are the hip, stifle, and hock. As these limbs consist of hinge joints which generally move in a cranial-to-caudal plane they enable alignment in this plane. Malalignment during fracture reduction, if modest, can be tolerated. Figure 1.20 illustrates how a modest malalignment can be tolerated in the case of caudal bending of a tibial fracture. The adjacent joints, the stifle and hock, are hinge joints and are held in somewhat 'compensatory' degrees of flexion or extension yielding minimal effect on total limb weight-bearing or gait. In some situations, this particular malalignment can provide stifle joint angulation similar to that seen following a Tibial Plateau Leveling Osteotomy (TPLO) to reposition the joint.

The extent to which a malalignment of the tibia or any other fractured long bone can be tolerated has not been studied. Malalignment should be avoided if at all possible but when it does occur in the cranial-caudal plane, it is more tolerated in the humerus, femur, and tibia. Radial and ulnar fractures seem to be less forgiving of cranial-caudal malalignment. Malalignment in the medial-lateral plane is critical. Malunion of this direction will result in valgus (outward angulation of the distal limb) or varus (inward angulation of the distal limb) deformity. Gait will be affected as will strain on the joints and other structures of the limb. Though the tolerable degree of malalignment in this plane has not be documented, all efforts should be made to accurately reduce the fracture in this plane.[41] If a postoperative radiograph demonstrates malalignment then the fracture fixation should promptly be revised. An exception may be in malalignment of the femur. Some malalignment may be tolerated, as the hip joint can accommodate this with some increase or decrease in the angle of inclination of the femoral head and neck. However, the severity of tolerable malalignment has not been described and should be kept minimal, or none at all, if possible.

Rotational alignment is inward or outward twisting of the distal limb. This too is not tolerated to any noticeable degree and will result in deleterious forces on the limb and an abnormal gait. The hinge joints of the limb generally function in a plane, and rotational malalignment places the joints out of that plane. Any appreciable malalignment must be corrected or revised in order to achieve proper limb function.

Apposition

Apposition refers to the closeness of fracture fragments. Absolute apposition may or may not be important, depending on the goal of the surgical technique. Biological repair of highly comminuted fractures is directed primarily to bone and limb alignment and not to apposition of all fracture lines. However, if a surgeon wishes to repair a limb in dynamic compression and there are fracture gaps, then load sharing, compression and dynamic

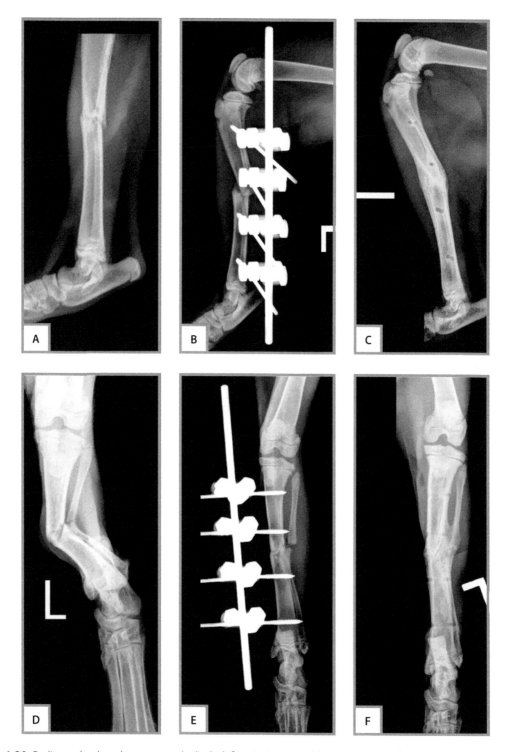

Figure 1.20 Radiographs show how an angular limb deformity is repaired by osteotomy, realignment and stabilization using a unilateral, Type I external fixator. Angular deformity in the medial-to-lateral plane is not tolerated and results in a valgus deformity and severe compromise to gait. Postoperatively, there is some angular malalignment in the cranial-to-caudal plane. Since the stifle and hock are hinges in this plane, there is no compromise to gait. (A) preoperative: lateral view; (B) postoperative: lateral view; (C) follow-up: lateral view (D) preoperative: dorsalplantar view; (E) postoperative: dorsalplantar view; (F) follow-up: dorsalplantar view.

compression will not be achieved, yielding results of high interfragmentary strain and potential complications. In general, if apposition is not achieved, there is the potential for deleterious consequences.

Apparatus

Apparatus is the evaluation of the repair construct in light of the device rules noted earlier. If the proper apparatus is used and applied using recommended methods then boney union is to be expected. Obeying all the rules is not always possible however, and despite that, healing may still occur. Fracture healing is directed by many dynamic influences. However, in evaluation of postoperative images, breaches in technique should be noted and the degree of influence on bone healing should be appraised. Specific issues to evaluate include whether implants have invaded joints or are of an inappropriate size or length. In follow-up radiographs, the implants should be evaluated for movement or loosening. Radiographic lucency around implants implies a loose implant and usually also implies instability and motion of the construct.

Activity

Activity refers to the healing noted on radiographic images. Of course, this is not a factor on immediate postoperative images. As a rule, bone healing is not apparent radiographically until after three weeks following an injury. However, an exception may be seen in very young patients as they tend to have more robust bone healing. Though exuberant healing may enhance the opportunity for boney union, a callus may have negative effects on limb function. An example is exuberant callus formation in distal femoral fractures of young patients. This can occur with Salter Harris fractures of the distal femur. Exuberant callus can incorporate the quadriceps muscle or entire quadriceps apparatus, resulting in quadriceps contractures/tie-down. This is a devastating complication that can usually be prevented with adequate fracture stabilization and postoperative physical therapy. In many situations bone healing occurs with minimal callus formation. In fractures where primary bone union is anticipated, such as with dynamic compression or in articular fractures, the fracture lines should become increasingly radiodense and less discernible over time with minimal callus formation. In these cases, lack of callus is desirable.

The amount of callus formation is also influenced by motion at the fracture site.[1] Increased motion will encourage callus formation as an endogenous biological method to stabilize the fracture. This is recognized as secondary bone union and often these fractures heal with an intermediate step of cartilage formation prior to endochondral ossification. Secondary bone union as a method of bone healing is often proper and desirable. However, the amount of motion at the fracture site may be too great and exceed the strain limits of healing bone-tissue. This results in a substitution of fibrous tissue formation and eventual non-union. Exuberant callus formation should be scrutinized and reimaged, as needed, to follow the progression of healing. If healing fails to progress, then additional interventions may be needed. There is an expected temporal progression of radiographic bone union. If secondary bone union is anticipated yet sufficient callus is not recognized radiographically, then one must accept that there are problems with the healing process and address the situation. Early callus formation is to be expected by three weeks following surgery. Bridging of the fracture callus should occur by six to eight weeks. Further maturation and remodeling of the fracture can take several months. If this progression does not occur, then ancillary procedures should be employed as appropriate. It is a mistake to refrain from intervention if secondary bone healing is anticipated yet no recognizable callus formation is present at six weeks. Rarely will waiting longer yield promising results, as the initial impetus for healing has subsided. It may be counterintuitive, but in fractures that are anticipated to take longer to heal, radiographs at an earlier stage may be helpful to track healing or document insufficient healing potential. Interventions can be initiated and, if needed, should be implemented sooner to shorten the overall healing time.

Radiolucent fracture lines may be seen between the original cortices in normal secondary bone healing. However, a bridging callus on the outside of the callus should be present by eight weeks. The outside of the fracture callus should be scrutinized in orthogonal views. A clearly discernible bridge should be seen in one or more parts of the bridging callus. If a bridging callus in at least one part of the callus is not seen by eight weeks, then a non-union is likely and intervention is warranted.

Complications

This book describes successful fracture repair techniques which are widely used. Complications are not presented in the case studies, but of course, complications do occur for even the most experienced surgeons. However, more often, complications occur from common mistakes that should be avoided.

Loose implants are, arguably, the most common cause of complication and often result in non-unions or the need for revision surgery. Non-secure implants which move damage healing tissues. The motion of fracture fragments, when greater than the tolerable strain of healing tissues, will not allow bone union and can predispose fibrous tissue formation.[42] If cartilage forms as an intermediate step in bone healing, then endochondral ossification will transform the cartilage into bone. However, fibrous tissue does not simply transform into bone. The formation of fibrous tissue due to the motion of implants, or motion of fracture fragments within the fracture site is a severe complication that must be avoided.

Improper application of cerclage wire is a frequently reported cause of non-unions. Cerclage wire must be applied according to the rules described and must stay tight throughout bone healing. Any cerclage wire that is noted to be loose, at any time, must be removed or replaced. Wires will not become tight with further healing. Many different cerclage wire techniques have been described including hemi-cerclage and different figure-of-eight configurations. Cerclage wire configurations are often placed in the area of bone healing and if they become loose, then healing is disrupted. It is best to avoid the use of cerclage wire except as described.

Improper use of IM pins is also a commonly reported complication. Pins do not counter torsional forces and it is rare that the fracture configuration will adequately counter torsional loads. When not appropriately countered, motion occurs leading to high interfragmentary strain, and a non-union is very likely. In addition, if there is motion at the fracture site it is likely to result in movement of a pin. If a pin is observed to 'back out', then motion at the fracture site should be assumed and the fixation should be revised in such a way that the fracture is more adequately stabilized.

DCPs are relatively expensive and require considerable soft tissue exposure for application. It is a common mistake to use a shorter than appropriate plate to save cost, time, and exposure. Using a plate which is too short leads to the remaining ends of bone acting as lever arms on the plate and area of healing fracture. Plate loosening or screw failure can then result. These complications are avoided by using plates of a sufficient length.

Locking plates are relatively new to veterinary orthopedics and have unique mechanical properties, noted earlier. The most common complication resulting from locking plates is due to an insufficient number of screws being used on each side of the fracture.[28] As the screws are angle stable, weight-bearing will result in large loads at the plate/screw interface or the bone/screw interface. This can result in screw breakage or bone slicing. The application of sufficient numbers of screws or ancillary devices (plate/rod constructs, for example) to unload the locking plate and screws will avoid such issues.

External fixators have higher complication rates than other devices because the transfixation pins are placed into bone from outside the body. Soft tissues can become infected and pins can damage soft tissues upon placement. Infection around pins leads to compromise at the bone-pin interface and pin loosening. In most situations, an external fixator cannot be expected to stay secure in bone for longer than eight weeks. If fracture healing has not occurred by this time, then the fixator will not adequately support the healing bone and unwanted motion will increase leading most likely to non-union. Fixators of adequate stiffness must be used, the fixator must be properly monitored, and loose pins must be replaced prior to fracture healing.

Part 2

Clinical Cases

Open, Grade 1, Transverse Fracture of the Right Mandible

Signalment and History
An 11-year-old, neutered, female Chihuahua weighing 3.5 kg sustained a jaw fracture from a motor vehicle accident.

Patient Assessment
The patient was in good health for her age and had some dental tartar, but no dental disease affecting the alveolar pockets. Although there was bruising of the jaw and lacerations within the mouth, there were no other head injuries. Thoracic and abdominal radiographs were within normal limits. Mentation and cranial nerve examination were within normal limits. The patient was a good candidate for surgical repair. Without moderate or severe dental disease, jaw bone has a good blood supply and a favorable biologic environment for healing. Properly stabilized, the fracture has a good prognosis for healing.

Fracture Assessment
Grade 1 open transverse fracture of the body of the right mandible between the 3rd and 4th premolars, ventrally displaced 3 mm (Figures 2.1A–B). The fracture line may invade the alveolar sock of the 3rd premolar caudal root. Though the fracture is open and in a contaminated area (the mouth), grade I and II fractures of the jaw infrequently become infected, provided they maintain a good blood supply.
If there is considerable dental disease, the mandible can exhibit poor bone quality and be infection compromised. The overall oral health of this patient was good. The primary object of mandibular fracture repair is to restore alignment of dental occlusion. This priority supersedes interfragmentary apposition, especially in comminuted fractures. In order to assure reconstructed occlusion, it is often necessary to exteriorize an intraoperative endotracheal tube out through a pharyngeal incision so that the jaw can be closed in assessment.

Options for Repair Methods
Methods of repair can be divided into intraoral techniques, external fixation, and open reduction and internal fixation. Intraoral techniques include interdental wiring with inclusion of an acrylic splint. The advantage of these techniques is that a surgical approach can be avoided with the potential for compromising a tooth root. These acrylic devices often become odorous and require removal under anesthesia and the teeth cleaned and polished.

External fixators, specifically acrylic fixators, have been described for mandibular fractures. Although these techniques do not allow interfragmentary compression, they do allow greater freedom for pin placement so as to avoid tooth roots. These devices might also become odorous.

Open reduction and internal fixation techniques include cerclage wiring and bone plating. Wiring techniques are the less stable of the two and are less accurate for proper occlusion. Bone plates can either be dynamic compression or locking. Locking plates can offer greater stability for the thin mandibular bone and at the angle or vertical ramus. In addition, locking plates are not pressed to the bone which can affect alignment and occlusion when contouring is insufficient. Locking plates can also 'ride up' the bone to some degree.

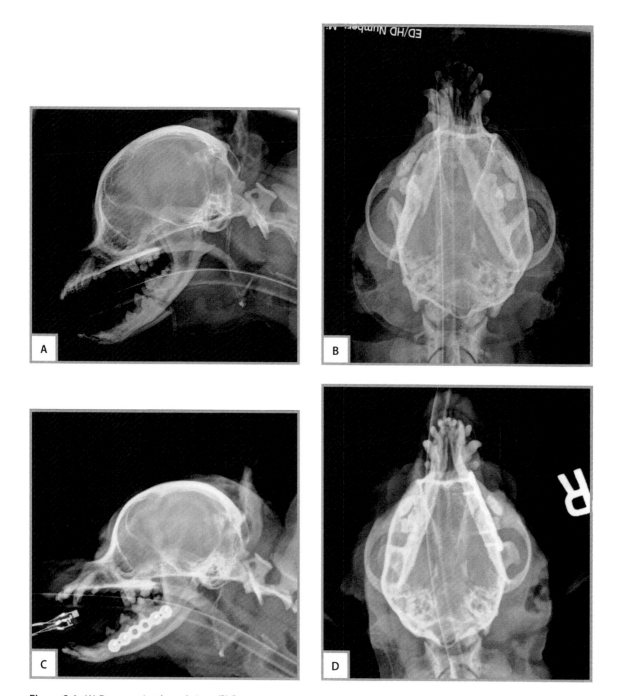

Figure 2.1 (A) Preoperative: lateral view; (B) Preoperative: caudal/rostral view; (C) Postoperative: lateral view; (D) Postoperative: caudal/rostral view.

(Continued)

Open, Grade 1, Transverse Fracture of the Right Mandible *continued*

Surgery Report

Preoperative planning was conducted to assure a plate selection which would avoid screw placement into tooth roots. The patient was placed in the dorsal recumbent position. An approach to the rostral shaft of the right hemimandible was performed. The fracture was reduced and a 6-hole locking plate was applied to the ventral mandibular ramus so that accompanying screws would best avoid tooth roots. Either tooth roots or fracture line infringement could not be avoided for screw holes 3 and 4 so they were left empty. The plate was minimally contoured and screws were placed in the order 5–3–6–1. The incision was closed routinely.

Postoperative Evaluation of Fracture Repair (Figures 2.1C–D)

Criteria	Assessment	Details
Alignment	Optimal	Radiographs, as well as postextubation observations, confirmed excellent dental occlusion.
Apposition	Optimal	The fracture line is not visible.
Apparatus	Good	There are only two screws both cranial and caudal to the fracture line. This was necessary to avoid tooth roots.

Follow-up at 6 Weeks (Figures 2.1E–F)

Criteria	Assessment
Alignment	Unchanged
Apposition	Unchanged
Apparatus	Unchanged
Activity	The fracture appears healed with minimal callus. There appears to be lucency around the tooth roots of the right 3rd and 4th premolars and the left lower canine. Dental cleaning and tooth extraction, as needed, were recommended.

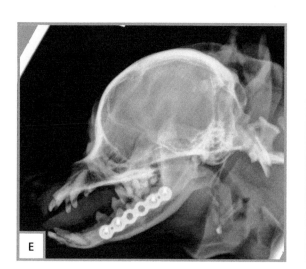

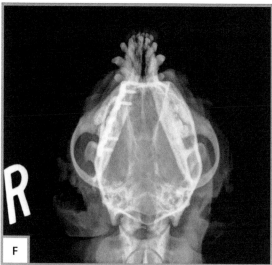

Figure 2.1 (Continued) (E) Follow-up at 6 Weeks: lateral view; (F) Follow-up at 6 Weeks: caudal/rostral view.

Closed, Transverse Fracture of the Left Scapula

Signalment and History

An 8-month-old, intact, female Golden Retriever weighing 23 kg sustained multiple traumatic injuries following a motor vehicle accident. She had been treated for shock, pneumothorax, rib fractures, left brachial plexus avulsion, and liver trauma. She was referred to the surgical referral hospital 14 days following the accident when a fractured scapula was diagnosed. At that time the patient was recovering well from the other injuries.

Patient Assessment

This was a very young patient with robust healing potential. Injuries aside from the scapula were healing and the patient's metabolic condition was good. Neurologic examination was within normal limits including sensation; suggesting normal function of the left brachial plexus. If there were a brachial plexus avulsion, the prognosis would be poor, as many, if not all, true brachial plexus avulsions do not recover to adequate function.

Fracture Assessment

Closed, transverse fracture of the glenoid and neck of the left scapula, proximally and medially displaced, and over-riding 4 mm (Figures 2.2A–B). The fracture was articular, which would suggest an internal fixation repair with accurate reduction and interfragmentary compression. The fracture was 14 days old and in this young dog, healing would already be underway. Reduction would be anticipated as difficult, and there may be cartilage damage, resulting in arthritis of the scapulohumeral joint.

Options for Repair Methods

Lag screw fixation of this fracture should be considered, as this would provide interfragmentary compression. Plate fixation with a DCP should also be considered because this would provide interfragmentary compression. This fracture was rather old and the patient was partially ambulating on this limb. Erosion of bone at the fracture line is likely to have occurred, making accurate and stable reduction difficult. In addition, the thin and soft scapular bone in this young animal is anticipated to give poor screw purchase when placed under compression. Locking plates would hold soft bone better, but would not provide compression across the articular fracture line.

Surgery Report

The patient was placed in the right lateral recumbent position and an approach to the body, spine, and acromion process of the scapula was performed. In order to expose the fracture, a partial elevation of the omotransversarious and acromial part of the deltoideus muscles was performed from the spine and acromion of the scapula. Fibrous tissue was removed from the fracture ends and the fracture was reduced and maintained in reduction with pointed reduction forceps. A 7-hole, 2.7 mm locking plate was contoured and applied to the scapula. The two most distal screws engaged the supraglenoid aspect of the fracture and the four proximal screws were positioned to penetrate the scapula at the angle of the spine and blade, taking advantage of dense bone at this location. Screw hole 5 was left open because of its location over a fracture line. The approach was closed routinely and the patient was placed in a spicca splint for 2 weeks.

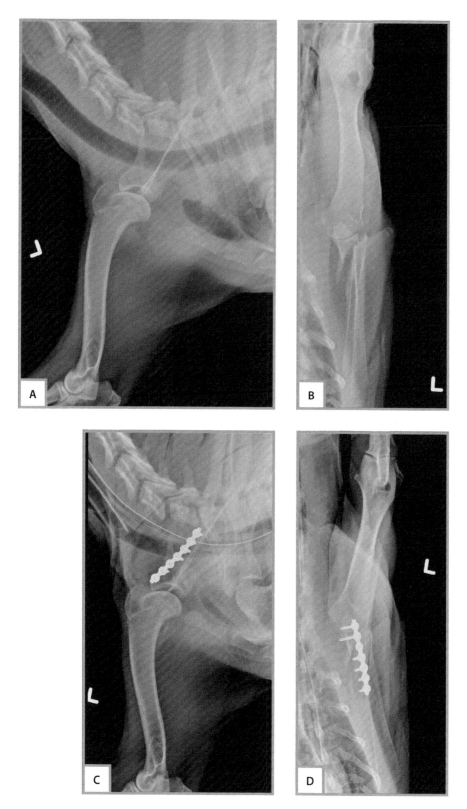

Figure 2.2 (A) Preoperative: lateral view; (B) Preoperative: cranial/caudal view; (C) Postoperative: lateral view; (D) Postoperative: cranial/caudal view.

(Continued).

Closed, Transverse Fracture of the Left Scapula *continued*

Postoperative Evaluation of Fracture Repair (Figures 2.2C–D)

Criteria	Assessment	Details
Alignment	Sufficient	There is a small step in the contour of the glenoid and a malformation to the shape of the glenoid, validating that the fracture was not (could not be) anatomically reduced.
Apposition	Sufficient	There appears to be good apposition at the fracture line.
Apparatus	Sufficient	There are two screws in the distal segment of the neck and glenoid. With a locking plate, more screws per bone segment would be preferable, but this could not be accomplished due to the size of the fragment. A lag screw could not be used, as it may interfere with those screws of the plate. In addition, the fracture did not anatomically reduce, resulting in questionable fixation stability. The proximal screws were placed close to the spine of the scapula to engage thicker bone.

Follow-up at 6 Weeks (Figures 2.2E–F)

Criteria	Assessment
Alignment	There appears to be improved contour of the glenoid.
Apposition	Unchanged
Apparatus	Unchanged
Activity	The fracture lines are no longer visible. There is minimal callus apparent in this image. The patient was allowed a slow return to activity.

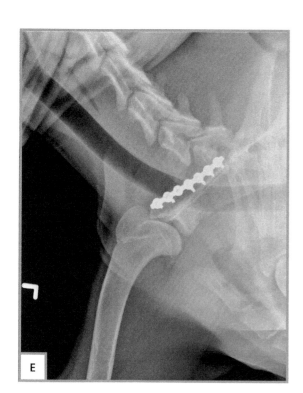

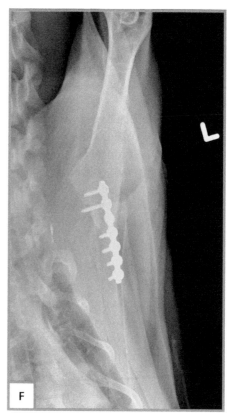

Figure 2.2 (Continued) (E) Follow-up at 6 Weeks: lateral view; (F) Follow-up at 6 Weeks: cranial/caudal view.

Closed, Short Oblique Fracture of the Humeral Condyle

Signalment and History
A 1.5-year-old, neutered, female Golden Retriever weighing 22 kg sustained right forelimb and right caudal limb fractures from a motor vehicle accident. The patient was initially treated with pain medications and intravenous fluids. Thoracic and abdominal radiographs were within normal limits. Neurologic examination was within normal limits.

Patient Assessment
This is a polytrauma case where soft tissue damage and increased risk of complications are frequent. Contributing to the risk of infection are increased anesthesia times for reparative surgery. This is a young, healthy patient with robust potential for healing. For simplicity, only the humeral fracture will be discussed.

Fracture Assessment
Closed, short oblique fracture of the distal 4th of the humeral condyle with a 2.5 cm by 1 cm butterfly fragment. Fractures of the humeral diaphysis are often difficult to repair due to the challenges of surgical approach and the required management of the large and complex forces placed on the humerus during postoperative ambulation. Of particular note is that the patient must carry additional weight-bearing on the fractured humerus as there is also a fracture of the ipsilateral caudal limb (Figures 2.3A–B).

Options for Repair Methods
External fixators would not be an appropriate choice. Unilateral fixators are not sufficiently strong and conventional bilateral fixators are not an option for fractures above the elbow (or above the stifle). An IM tie-in configuration could be considered, but such a construct may still not be strong enough and the external apparatus is difficult to maintain.

An interlocking IM nail is also not a suitable choice, as the distal fragment could not accommodate two distal screws.

Plate fixation with either a DCP or locking plate should be considered. A locking plate, especially those that can be contoured to the epicondylar ridges would be appropriate. Configurations might include two lateral plates; one positioned on the lateral epicondylar ridge and one medially. This would allow adequate screw purchase in the distal segment. Mechanically, plates on the medial and lateral epicondylar ridges would be better.

Alternatively, a medial plate, either locking or dynamic compression, could be used. A medial plate could be applied in dynamic compression or load sharing, although access to the butterfly segment would be more difficult.

Surgery Report
The patient was placed in the left lateral recumbent position and an approach to the distal shaft of the humerus through a craniolateral incision was performed. The butterfly fragment was reduced to the proximal segment and maintained in reduction with pointed reduction-forceps. The fragment was then stabilized with two 2.7 mm screws placed in lag fashion. A 2.7 mm cortical screw was applied in lag fashion to secure the fragment to the proximal segment. The remaining two fracture segments were reduced using Kern bone-holding forceps. A 12-hole 2.7 mm locking plate was contoured to the craniolateral aspect of the humerus. One screw was placed proximally in hole 2 followed by insertion of a screw distally in hole 10. The remaining screws were inserted, excepting in holes 4 and 8. Care was taken not to enter the olecranon fossa of the distal humerus. A second 12-hole 2.7 mm locking plate was contoured and applied caudal to, but paralleling, the first. Holes 4, 7, and 8 were left open.

A bone graft was obtained from the proximal humerus and applied to the medial fracture lines. The incision was closed routinely.

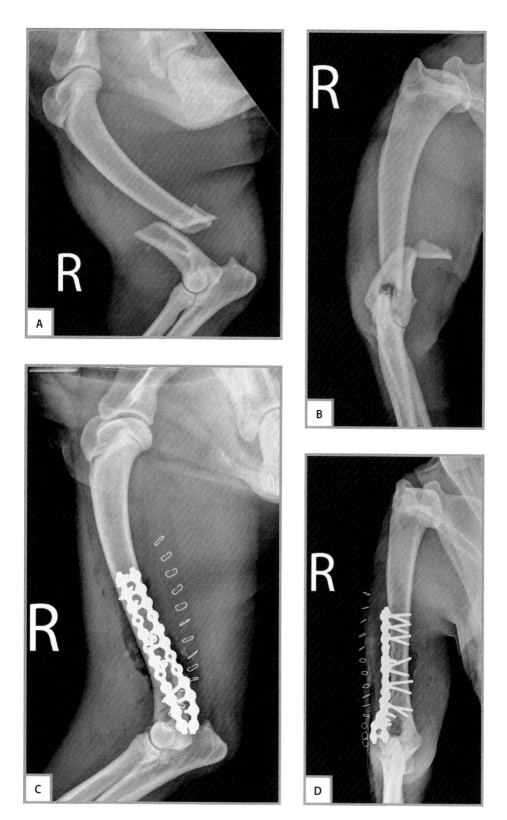

Figure 2.3 (A) Preoperative: lateral view; (B) Preoperative: cranial/caudal view; (C) Postoperative: lateral view; (D) Postoperative: cranial/caudal view.

(Continued)

Closed, Short Oblique Fracture of the Humeral Condyle *continued*

Postoperative Evaluation of Fracture Repair (Figures 2.3C–D)

Criteria	Assessment overview	Details
Alignment	Optimal	Anatomic reduction was achieved.
Apposition	Optimal	Interfragmentary compression was achieved across all fracture lines. Fracture lines could not be visualized on the medial cortex of the humerus suggesting that medial buttressing had been achieved.
Apparatus	Good	Although a single 2.7 mm plate would not be appropriate, pairing the plates was acceptable due to the shape of the plate. This increased the total number of screws on each side of the fracture and increased the AMI of the fixation construct. Placing a plate both medially and laterally would have provided greater fixation strength and stiffness, but also necessitated a trans-olecranon approach or a combined medial and lateral approach. Since a medial buttress was achieved with the use of lag screws, additional approaches were not necessary.

Follow-up at 9 Weeks (Figures 2.3E–F)

Criteria	Assessment
Alignment	Unchanged
Apposition	Unchanged
Apparatus	Unchanged
Activity	Callus has formed at the caudal, medial, and cranial cortical surfaces. The callus observed cranially appears elevated from the original cortex and may suggest fibrous tissue interference with bone growth or motion early in the healing process. The patient was slowly returned to normal activity.

Note: Case material supplied by Dr. Mary Sarah Bergh and Dr. Angell Thompson.

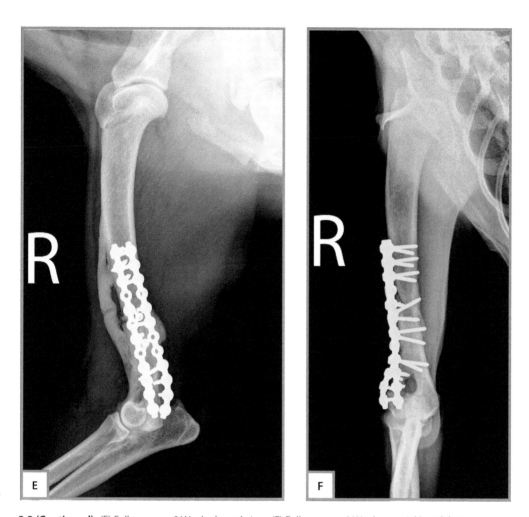

Figure 2.3 (Continued) (E) Follow-up at 9 Weeks: lateral view; (F) Follow-up at 9 Weeks: cranial/caudal view.

Closed, Salter IV Fracture of Lateral Humeral Condyle

Signalment and History

A 2-month-old, intact, female English Bulldog weighing 10 kg sustained an elbow fracture when jumping from its owner's arms the previous day.

Patient Assessment

This is a very young patient with soft, immature bones and considerable remaining growth potential.

Fracture Assessment

Closed, Salter IV fracture of the lateral humeral condyle, displaced laterally and over-riding 4 mm (Figures 2.4A–B).

Options for Repair Methods

This is an articular fracture and as such requires open reduction with rigid fixation and anatomic alignment. Transcondylar lag screw fixation with an additional anti-rotational supracondylar Kirschner wire is frequently used as fixation for these fractures. The fracture should be repaired as soon after injury as possible to prevent motion damaging soft bone and compromising a surgeon's ability to reduce the fracture. Potential problems from compromised growth at the distal physis and the development of osteoarthritis is a concern.

Surgery Report

An approach to the lateral aspect of the humeral condyle and epicondyle was performed. The extensor carpi radialis was elevated off the cranial aspect of the epicondylar ridge and the anconeus muscle was elevated off the caudal aspect. The fractured capitulum (lateral aspect of the humeral condyle) was reflected laterally, hinging on the collateral ligament until the fracture segment was exteriorized. A 4.0 mm drill bit was then used to drill a hole from the fracture line, in a lateral direction, but distal to the visualized physis. A cannula with an outer diameter of 3.5 mm and inner diameter of 2.5 mm was place from lateral-to-medial into this hole. This cannula was used for leverage to help reduce the fracture. The fracture was subsequently reduced so that the fracture line at the epicondylar ridge and the cranial articular surface could be confirmed for accurate reduction. Pointed reduction forceps were then used to stabilize the fracture. A 2.5 mm drill bit was used to drill through the cannula into the trochlea (medial aspect of the humeral condyle). The cannula was then removed. The drill hole was measured and a screw slightly shorter than this measurement was chosen for placement to assure the screw did not protrude too far on the medial aspect of the condyle when seated into the lateral collateral ligament. A washer was also used with this screw, after considering the softness of this immature bone. A 4.0 mm tap was used to tap the medial aspect of the condyle, after which a 4.0 mm cancellous screw wish washer was placed in lag fashion. A 1.1 mm (17 gauge) Kirschner wire was drilled from the lateral epicondyle, up the epicondylar ridge and exited the medial aspect of the distal humeral metaphysis, with care taken to avoid entry into the supratrochlear foramen/olecranon fossa. The extensor carpi radialis was sutured to the anconeus muscle, followed by routine closure.

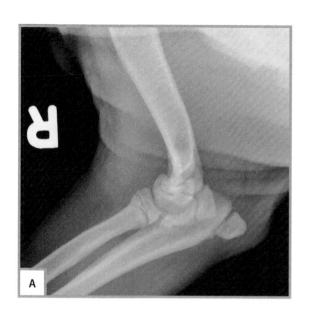

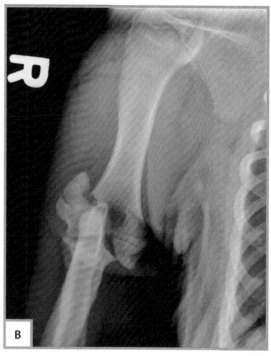

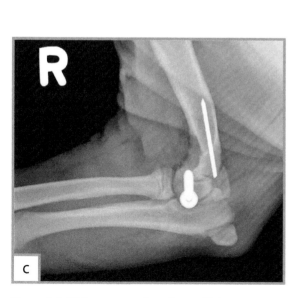

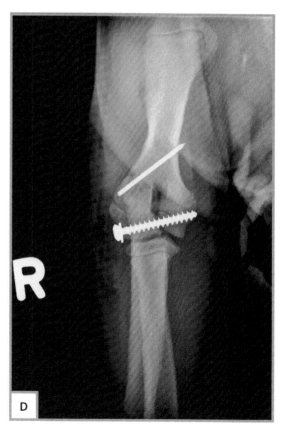

Figure 2.4 (A) Preoperative: lateral view; (B) Preoperative: cranial/caudal view; (C) Postoperative: lateral view; (D) Postoperative: cranial/caudal view.

(Continued)

Closed, Salter IV Fracture of Lateral Humeral Condyle *continued*

Postoperative Evaluation of Fracture Repair (Figures 2.4C–D)

Criteria	Assessment	Details
Alignment	Sufficient	There is a small step at the articular surface. This may have resulted from soft bone collapse during lagging.
Apposition	Sufficient	The fracture line is visible and there seems to be a small gap. The epicondyle appears to be anatomically reduced.
Apparatus	Good	The screw appears to be placed below the physis and across the condyle. The Kirschner wire is appropriately placed up the epicondyle.

Follow-up at 7 Weeks (Figures 2.4E–F)

Criteria	Assessment
Alignment	The step in the articular surface, seen postoperatively, is not present and appears to have remodeled.
Apposition	The fracture line is no longer visible.
Apparatus	The screw and wire are basically unchanged in position. There appears to be some lucency around the washer.
Activity	Minimal callus formation is present. The fracture lines of the condyle and epicondylar ridge are no longer apparent. The condylar physis appears to be closed and the condyle has a normal appearance. There was good range of motion. The patient was allowed to return to normal activity.

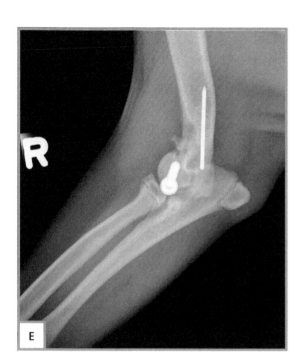

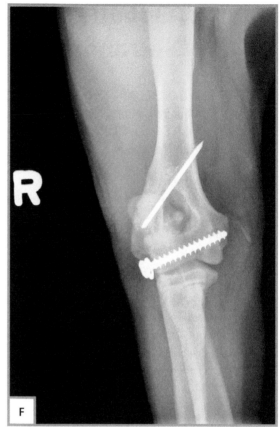

Figure 2.4 (Continued) (E) Follow-up at 7 Weeks: lateral view; (F) Follow-up at 7 Weeks: cranial/caudal view.

Closed, Oblique, Articular Fracture of the Olecranon

Signalment and History
A 7-year-old, neutered, male Labrador Retriever Mix weighing 43 kg sustained a left forelimb injury from a motor vehicle accident.

Patient Assessment
The patient was admitted in generally good health. Thoracic and abdominal radiographs were within normal limits. The forelimb had not sustained severe soft tissue damage. Although an older patient, there should be no compromise to healing potential.

Fracture Assessment
Closed, oblique, articular fracture of the olecranon, proximally displaced less than 5 mm. One small, single fragment comminution at the distal fracture line is present (Figures 2.5A–B).

Options for Repair Methods
External support would not be appropriate due to the distracting pull of the triceps, the fracture being articular and the proximal location of the fracture in the ulna. The olecranon is under tension from the triceps. As such, a method which includes a tension device should be chosen to redirect tensile forces into compressive forces. The fracture was also articular, therefore it must be anatomically reduced at the articular surface. A tension-band device with pins and cerclage wire would be an option, but it is difficult to position these devices so that the pins reduce the fracture properly and stay rigid. The proximal pins and cerclage wire must be positioned so that they do not impinge the triceps tendon. Plate fixation, preferably with dynamic compression, could be performed; and, if positioned sufficiently caudal, could act as a tension-band device resulting in compression.

Surgery Report
The patient was placed in the dorsal recumbent position and an approach to the tuber olecranon was performed. The fracture was reduced and a 7-hole locking plate applied to the lateral aspect of the ulna. Screws were applied in buttress fashion in the order 2–6–1–3–5–7.

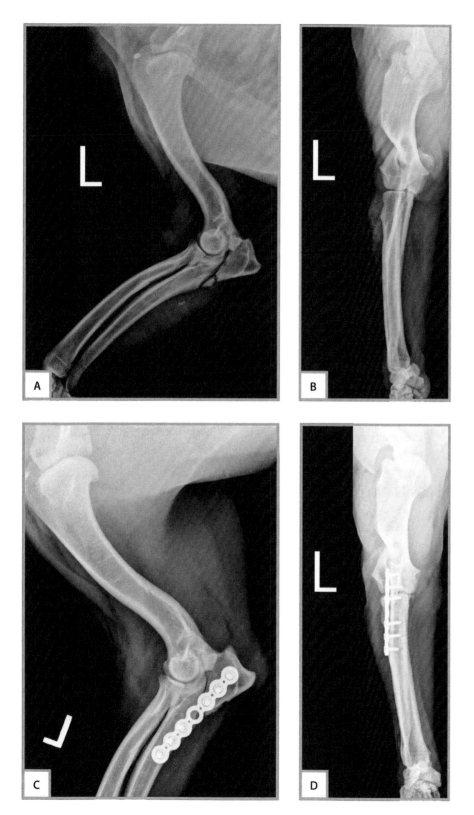

Figure 2.5 (A) Preoperative: lateral view; (B) Preoperative: cranial/caudal view; (C) Postoperative: lateral view; (D) Postoperative: cranial/caudal view.

(Continued)

Closed, Oblique, Articular Fracture of the Olecranon *continued*

Postoperative Evaluation of Fracture Repair (Figures 2.5C–D)

Criteria	Assessment	Details
Alignment	Good	The fracture was anatomically aligned.
Apposition	Insufficient	A fracture gap can be seen at the articular surface. A fragment of (comminuted) bone has been removed from the caudal-distal aspect of the fracture line.
Apparatus	Sufficient	A locking plate was selected that holds the bone fragments in position and provides buttress support to the fracture. The olecranon is under tension from the pull of the triceps. It should be noted that unless the plate is sufficiently caudal and elastic, and the fracture line is allowed to undergo compression, the plate may cause high interfragmentary strain on the small fracture gap observed. This can lead to delayed union and shear stress, depending on the pull of the triceps.

First Follow-up at 7 Weeks (Figures 2.5E–F)

Criteria	Assessment
Alignment	Unchanged
Apposition	The fracture line is more distinct especially at the articular surface.
Apparatus	Unchanged
Activity	There is little callus present. This is probably due to high interfragmentary strain with the plate insufficiently acting as a tension-band device. The implants are stable and there may be some areas of bridging bone close to the plate. If there is a boney bridge, then the fracture is likely to heal.

Final Follow-up at 12 Weeks (Figures 2.5G–H)

Criteria	Assessment
Alignment	Unchanged
Apposition	Unchanged
Apparatus	Unchanged
Activity	Although the fracture line can be seen, there appears to be bridging bone throughout the fracture line, excepting the distal most aspect of the fracture line, which had a bone fragment removed. The patient was slowly returned to normal activity.

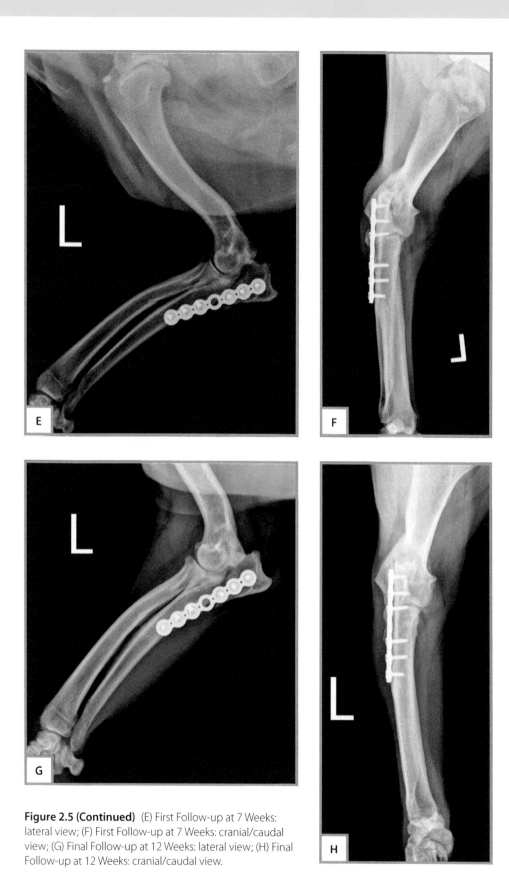

Figure 2.5 (Continued) (E) First Follow-up at 7 Weeks: lateral view; (F) First Follow-up at 7 Weeks: cranial/caudal view; (G) Final Follow-up at 12 Weeks: lateral view; (H) Final Follow-up at 12 Weeks: cranial/caudal view.

Closed, Transverse Fracture of the Right Radius and Ulna

Signalment and History
A 3-year-old, neutered, male Yorkshire Terrier weighing 4.5 kg sustained a fracture to the right radius and ulna whilst playing with other dogs.

Patient Assessment
This is a relatively young dog, but it is a miniature breed known to be at risk of delayed healing of fractures to the radius and ulna.

Fracture Assessment
Closed, transverse fracture of the distal 3rd of the right radius and ulna, angularly displaced cranially but not over-riding (Figures 2.6A–B). Please note in human medicine, the term *Colles' Fracture* describes a fracture at the distal end of the radius.

Options for Repair Methods
Fractures of the radius and ulna in miniature breed dogs are often transverse and can occur from minimal trauma due to the small size of the bone and small AMI. There is also scant soft tissue coverage, small IM space and low biological activity. As such, primary bone union would be preferred. With secondary bone union, the biological environment is challenged to establish a callus. Because primary bone union is the goal, dynamic compression plating would be a first choice. All efforts should be made to place the plate in dynamic compression so as to allow axial load-bearing during the healing period. Other plating techniques could be considered such as cuttable plates or plates acting in buttress, including locking plates. External fixation techniques, such as ring fixators, can be successfully used in such cases, although complications are common. External support with a cast or splint is not recommended. Casts/splints do not provide sufficiently rigid fixation for primary bone union and they suppress secondary bone union. Non-unions are frequent when external support is utilized. When considering internal plate fixation, all efforts should be made to engage six bone cortices with screws on each side of the fracture. Fractures can be very distal, allowing only four cortices of purchase, which is not optimal. However, in some cases, there are no alternatives. T-plates can be used to allow the maximum number of distal cortices in very distal fractures. Bone grafting is also recommended.

Surgery Report
The patient was placed in the dorsal recumbent position and a 1 cm incision was made over the greater tubercle of the right humerus in order to harvest a bone graft. The outer cortex was penetrated with a 3.2 mm Steinmann pin. A 3-0 curette was used to remove cancellous bone which was transferred to a syringe barrel. Approximately 0.25 ml of cancellous bone was obtained. This incision was closed. An approach to the shaft of the radius through a medial incision was made. The fracture was reduced and a 7-hole, 2.0 mm LC-DCP plate was contoured to the cranial aspect of the radius. Upon observing cortical contact on the caudal aspect of the radius, a slight pre-bend of the plate enabled the plate to rise above the fracture line by approximately 0.5 mm. A 2.0 mm screw was positioned into screw hole 5. That screw was inserted loosely so that the plate could slide cranially. A 2nd screw was then inserted under dynamic compression into hole 3. This effectively loaded one screw on each side of the fracture. Subsequent screws were inserted in sequence proximal to distal. The cancellous graft was placed caudal to the radius and the wound closed routinely.

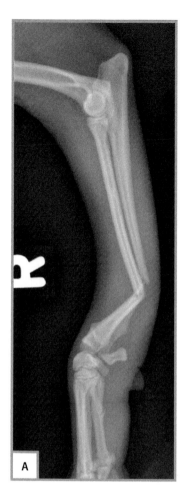

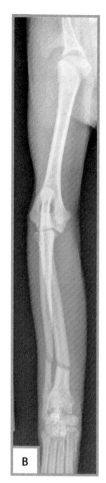

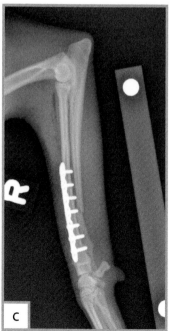

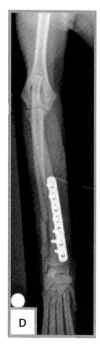

Figure 2.6 (A) Preoperative: lateral view; (B) Preoperative: cranial/caudal view; (C) Postoperative: lateral view; (D) Postoperative: cranial/caudal view. *(Continued)*

Closed, Transverse Fracture of the Right Radius and Ulna *continued*

Postoperative Evaluation of Fracture Repair (Figures 2.6C–D)

Criteria	Assessment Overview	Details
Alignment	Optimal	The fracture is anatomically aligned.
Apposition	Optimal	The fracture line is compressed and not visible.
Apparatus	Good	The plate has been appropriately attached with compression of the 3rd and 5th screws. The plate could perhaps have been longer, with one more distal and one more proximal hole. The proximal limit of the applied plate is mid-radius. Depending on the stiffness of the plate compared to the stiffness of the bone, this proximal plate location could be a stress-riser. In small dogs, the choice of plate for optimal stiffness is not straightforward. If the plate is too stiff, the healing bone will be stress-protected; leading to delayed healing and osteoporosis. If the plate is insufficiently stiff, then the plate may fail. This can be due to plate bending or cyclic failure and plate breakage. The plate selected in this case appears to be appropriate for this patient.

Follow-up at 7 Weeks (Figures 2.6E–F)

Criteria	Assessment
Alignment	Unchanged
Apposition	Unchanged
Apparatus	Unchanged
Activity	The fracture line is not visible and appears healed. However, the ulna has not healed and appears to be progressing to non-union. This is not of clinical concern unless it is causing the patient pain. At this time it cannot be determined if the plate is too stiff although it is thought unlikely that a 2.0 mm plate would be too stiff given the size of the patient. If the plate is stress-protecting the fracture, then with the passage of time, the radius will become osteopenic. It is recommended that the limb is radiographed at 6-month intervals to follow the course of the remodeling. If the radius becomes osteopenic, then staged plate removal would be recommended.

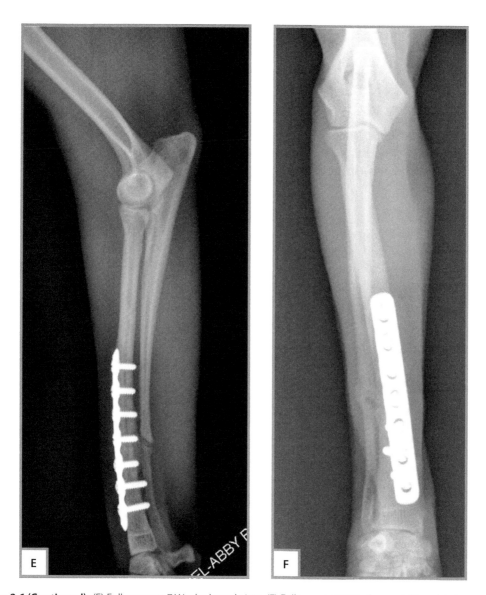

Figure 2.6 (Continued) (E) Follow-up at 7 Weeks: lateral view; (F) Follow-up at 7 Weeks: cranial/caudal view.

Closed, Transverse Fracture of the Left Radius and Ulna

Signalment and History

A 9-year, 8-month-old, neutered, female German Shepherd weighing 45 kg sustained a left radius and ulna fracture from a low-speed motor vehicle accident (snow machine).

Patient Assessment

Though almost 10 years old, the patient was in good general health. Thoracic and abdominal radiographs were within normal limits, as were other physical parameters. A splint was placed soon after the incident.

Fracture Assessment

On palpation, the limb was not unduly swollen or unstable. Forelimb radiographs revealed a closed, transverse fracture of the distal 4th of the left radius and ulna, displaced laterally and over-riding 1 cm (Figures 2.7A–B).

Options for Repair Methods

This transverse, non-comminuted fracture is an excellent candidate for a DCP. The fracture is reducible, not comminuted, and will allow true dynamic compression if the plate is applied appropriately. Primary bone union would be expected in the radius. The ulna is not weight-bearing and in most cases is not repaired.

IM pinning, casting, or locking nail fixation would be far less appropriate. Buttress fixation with a locking plate or external fixator could be effective, but would not be a primary choice as these fixation devices do not usually allow dynamic compression and are less able to allow axial loads to compress the fracture line with load sharing. High interfragmentary strain may occur with such buttress types of fixation.

Though osteosynthesis would be expected with dynamic plate fixation, healing may be delayed due to the age of the patient and fracture location at the distal antebrachium; an area of relatively low vascular support. For this reason bone grafting should be considered, but might not be considered critical in this larger size of dog.

Surgery Report

An autogenous cancellous bone graft was obtained from the proximal humerus of the same limb. An approach to the shaft of the radius through a medial incision was performed. The fracture was reduced using Kern bone-holding forceps. An 8-hole, 3.5 mm LC-DCP broad plate was contoured to the dorsal aspect of the radius. The plate was then pre-bent between screw holes 5 and 6 so that the plate was elevated 1 mm above the radius at the fracture site. A screw was inserted into hole 7 first, but not tightened completely. The plate was then slipped proximally, so that the screw came to reside in the distal aspect of the dynamic compression hole, i.e., eccentrically (loaded). The screw inserted into hole 4 was applied with dynamic compression and the screw in hole 7 was then tightened. This effectively resulted in screws placed with compression on each side of the fracture, yielding compression of the trans-cortex as the pre-bent plate was secured to the radius. The remaining screws were placed, but not in compression. The bone graft was placed on the palmar aspect of the fracture site.

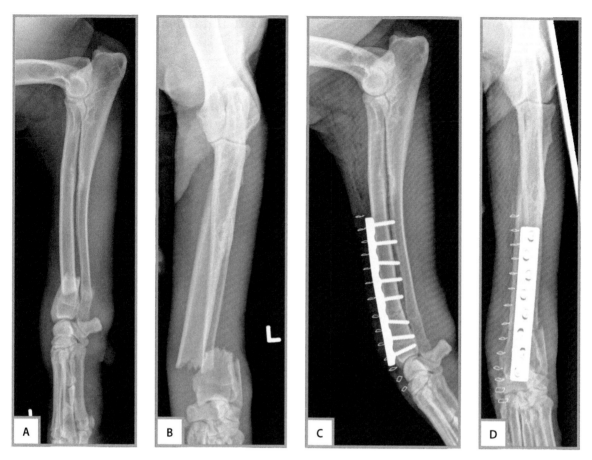

Figure 2.7 (A) Preoperative: lateral view; (B) Preoperative: cranial/caudal view; (C) Postoperative: lateral view; (D) Postoperative: cranial/caudal view.

(Continued)

Closed, Transverse Fracture of the Left Radius and Ulna *continued*

Postoperative Evaluation of Fracture Repair (Figures 2.7C–D)

Criteria	Assessment Overview	Details
Alignment	Optimal	This simple fracture was anatomically reduced; restoring alignment in all planes and neutralizing torsion.
Apposition	Optimal	All fracture lines appear to have complete contact closure.
Apparatus	Optimal	The plate was applied according to guidelines with at least three screws engaging 6 cortices in the distal bone segment. The plate is close to the radial carpal joint, which may result in discomfort.

Follow-up at 8 Weeks (Figures 2.7E–F)

Criteria	Assessment
Alignment	Unchanged
Apposition	Unchanged
Apparatus	Unchanged
Activity	There is increased sclerosis and healing at the fracture site and some new bone proliferation at both the palmar and medial aspects of the radius. This suggests mostly primary bone union, but with some callus; probably due to the bone graft. There is evidence of bridging callus formation of the ulna, suggesting secondary bone union of the ulna.

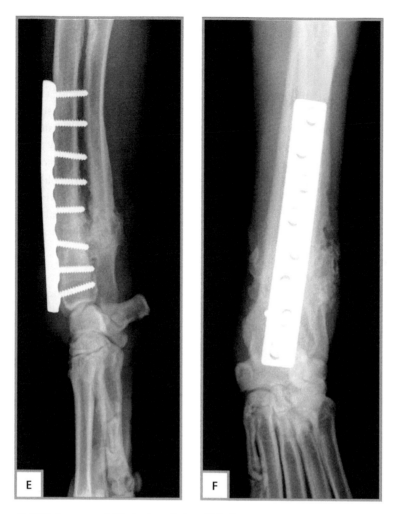

Figure 2.7 (Continued) (E) Follow-up at 8 Weeks: lateral view; (F) Follow-up at 8 Weeks: caudal/cranial view.

Closed, Salter II Fracture of the Distal Radius

Signalment and History
An 8-month-old, castrated, male Siberian Husky weighing 24 kg sustained a fracture to the right radius and ulna at a boarding facility. Both closed and open reduction were unsuccessfully attempted at a primary care facility. The patient was presented to the referral hospital 1 week after injury.

Patient Assessment
The patient is young and may have additional growth potential at the distal radial and ulnar physes. The fracture has been previously operated, increasing the chance of infection, and cultures should be taken during surgery.

Fracture Assessment
Closed Salter II fracture of the distal radius, displaced cranially. The distal ulna appears normal; however, premature closure is a possibility. Though the fracture is somewhat stable, it places the radial carpal joint in an abnormal position. Trauma to the physes of the distal antebrachium could lead to angular limb deformity (Figures 2.8A–B).

Options for Repair Methods
Cross pins have been used in the treatment of this type of fracture, but would be an inferior stand-alone choice. Plate fixation would be stiffer and stronger, but the distal radial epiphysis offers a restricted amount of bone stock for screw purchase. Accordingly, a T-plate can be used.

Available T-plates are relatively thin and therefore rather weak if bending is required. In the event of distal-radial physeal closure from plate fixation in the face of continued distal-ulnar physeal growth, a distal-ulnar osteotomy may be warranted to prevent angular limb deformity. This would place additional load on the plate. A combination of plate and cross-pin fixation would enhance fixation strength. Canine femoral hook-plate fixation has also been used in this type of fracture and described.

Surgery Report
An approach to the distal ulna was performed. The periosteum of the ulna was elevated and a 1 cm section removed just proximal to the distal physis using a pneumatic saw. An approach to the distal radius through a dorsal approach was performed. The fracture was reduced using a periosteal elevator. Two 1.6 mm (0.062 inch) Kirschner wires were driven from the styloid processes of the radius across the fracture at approximately 45 degree angles. A 9-hole 3.5 mm T-plate was applied to the dorsal surface of the radius. Two 4.0 mm cancellous screws were placed distally, paralleling the radial-carpal joint. Seven 3.5 mm cortical screws were used for the proximal holes. The 4.0 mm cancellous screws were placed first to assure that the plate was adequately positioned proximally. Thereafter, the remaining cortical screws were placed.

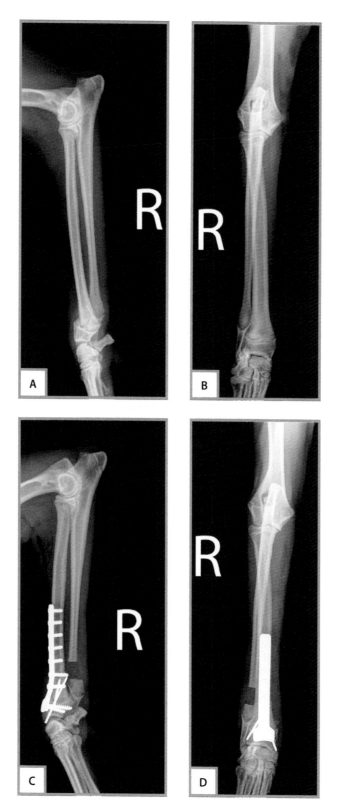

Figure 2.8 (A) Preoperative: lateral view; (B) Preoperative: cranial/caudal view; (C) Postoperative: lateral view; (D) Postoperative: cranial/caudal view.

(Continued)

Closed, Salter II Fracture of the Distal Radius *continued*

Postoperative Evaluation of Fracture Repair (Figures 2.8C–D)

Criteria	Assessment	Details
Alignment	Good	The fracture was slightly over-reduced, but the proximal and distal articular surfaces of the radial-carpal joint appear parallel.
Apposition	Optimal	The fracture line appears compressed.
Apparatus	Optimal	The pins, plate, and screws were correctly positioned.

First Follow-up at 12 Weeks (Figures 2.8E–F)

Criteria	Assessment
Alignment	Unchanged
Apposition	Unchanged
Apparatus	Unchanged
Activity	The follow-up radiographs were taken later than requested. The fracture line appears completely healed with little callus formation. The defect in the distal ulna has completely filled. There is sclerosis and new bone formation at the proximal aspect of the bone plate; apparently a response to increased stresses associated with a riser due to the plate. For this reason, plate removal was proposed and performed.

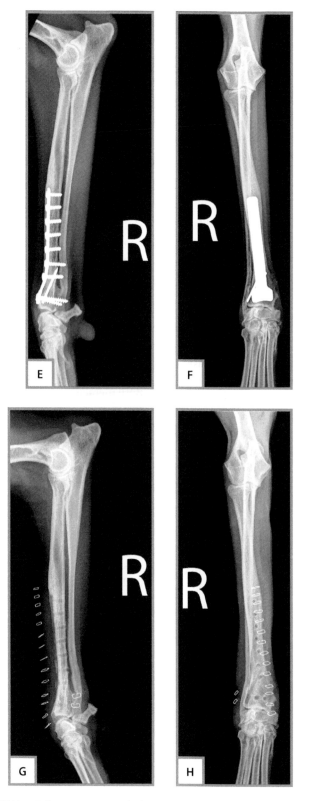

Figure 2.8 (Continued) (E) First Follow-up at 12 Weeks: lateral view; (F) First Follow-up at 12 Weeks: cranial/caudal view; (G) Post plate removal: lateral view (H) Post plate removal cranial/caudal view.

Closed, Transverse, Mid-Diaphyseal Fractures of Metacarpals

Signalment and History
A 2-year-old, neutered, female mixed-breed weighing 35 kg presented for injury sustained to the left metacarpals from a farm implement accident.

Patient Assessment
There were numerous abrasions on the left antebrachium and carpal area. Otherwise, the patient was in good physical condition.

Fracture Assessment
Closed, transverse, mid-diaphyseal fractures of metacarpals 2, 3, 4, and 5 displaced caudally and overriding up to 8 mm (Figures 2.9A–B).

Options for Repair Methods
Although there were numerous superficial abrasions, none communicated with the fractures. External support with a non-weight-bearing device such as a cast or spoon splint should be considered if one or more metacarpal bones are intact, the fractures are not significantly displaced and the biological environment is deemed adequate. Otherwise, internal fixation should be recommended. Intramedullary pinning is one such technique involving small Kirschner wires inserted into holes drilled in the distal ends of the metacarpals. The wires are then advanced proximally across the fracture site. The holes should be rather large as wires are prone to penetrating the palmar cortex. A toggle-pinning technique can be used where Kirschner wires are placed distally, then cut 3–4 mm long. The proximal metacarpal segments are toggled onto those protruding segments of pins. Both of these techniques are tenuous and although often successful, they do frequently fail and therefore need to be supported with a cast or splint. Plating of the metacarpal bone provides support and allows early weight-bearing. The major disadvantage is the approach and the cost of implants are much greater than pinning techniques. Regardless of the technique, applying fixation devices to all fractured metacarpals is recommended as multiple fixations support one another.

Surgery Report
A dorsal, linear incision was made the length of the metacarpals between metacarpals 4 and 5. Both metacarpal (MC) bones were exposed with a periosteal elevator. The fractures were reduced and 2.0 mm LC-DCP plates were applied to the dorsal surfaces. A 7-hole plate was applied to MC5 with three screws proximal to the fracture and four screws distal. All screws were placed in neutral fashion. A 6-hole plate was applied to MC4. A second incision was made between MC2 and MC3. A 5-hole plate was applied to MC2 with two screws proximal to the fracture and a 6-hole plate was applied to MC3 with three screws proximal to the fracture. The incision was closed routinely. A padded bandage was maintained for 2 weeks.

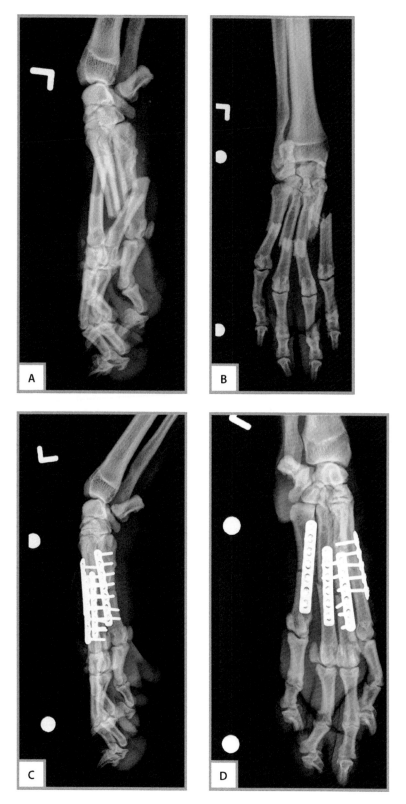

Figure 2.9 (A) Preoperative: lateral view; (B) Preoperative: dorsalpalmer view; (C) Postoperative: lateral view; (D) Postoperative: dorsalpalmer view. *(Continued)*

Closed, Transverse, Mid-Diaphyseal Fractures of Metacarpals *continued*

Postoperative Evaluation of Fracture Repair (Figures 2.9C–D)

Criteria	Assessment	Details
Alignment	Optimal	The metacarpals were anatomically reduced and aligned.
Apposition	Good	There are visible fracture lines and subtle translation of fractures at MC3, 4, and 5.
Apparatus	Sufficient	Only two screws were placed proximal to the fracture in MC2. Though this was due to having insufficient numbers of 6-hole plates available, a longer 7-hole plate should have been chosen. The 3rd screw from proximal appears too close to the fracture line in MC3 and MC4. The LC-DCP plate should have been applied in dynamic compression, placing the screws eccentrically in the screw holes away from the fracture. This would have offered compression, better apposition, and would have placed those screws at the fracture line farther from the fracture.

Follow-up at 5 Weeks (Figures 2.9E–F)

Criteria	Assessment
Alignment	Unchanged
Apposition	Unchanged
Apparatus	Unchanged
Activity	Good, there is minimal callus at all healing metacarpals. The patient was slowly returned to normal activity.

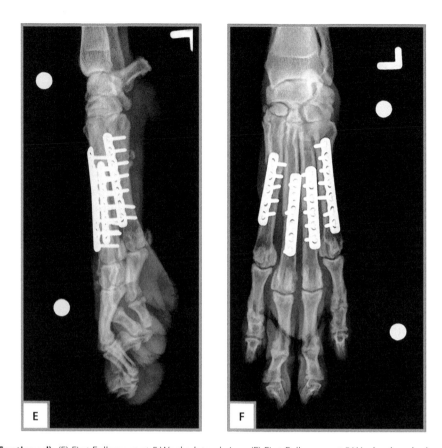

Figure 2.9 (Continued) (E) First Follow-up at 5 Weeks: lateral view; (F) First Follow-up at 5 Weeks: dorsalpalmer view.

Closed, Fracture/Luxation of the T12–13 Vertebrae

Signalment and History

An 18-month-old, castrated, male Shetland Sheep dog weighing 22 kg sustained a spinal cord injury following a motor vehicle accident. The patient was presented to an emergency clinic non-ambulatory in the caudal limb. Dexamethasone and butorphanol was administered prior to referral to a surgical hospital.

Patient Assessment

The patient was not ambulatory. Cranial nerve examination was within normal limits. Forelimb sensation and motor function was normal, but appeared to extend forelimbs rigidly. Paniculus reflex was lost at the T13–L1 area. There was no purposeful motor function of the caudal limbs. Patellar and cranial tibial reflexes were normal to hyper-reflexive. Anal reflex was present. Crossed extensor reflex was present and hyper-reflexic. Pain sensation was present on the medial (femoral innervations) and lateral (sciatic innervations) aspect of the caudal limb. Thoracic and abdominal radiographs were within normal limits. The patient was obese with a body condition score of 8/9. This may complicate surgery and reduce speed of recovery, but not overall prognosis.

The presence or absence of deep pain sensation is an important prognostic indicator in traumatic spinal cord injury in dogs. If deep pain is present and caudal limb reflexes suggest upper motor signs, prognosis for ambulation and normal urinary and fecal continence is good. If there is no conscious recognition of painful stimuli, and deep pain sensation is not present then prognosis is poor for return of caudal limb neurologic function.

Fracture Assessment

Closed fracture/luxation of the T12-13 vertebrae, ventrally luxated 3 mm with fracture of the T13 endplate and fracture of left transitional vertebrae (Figures 2.4A–B). Note: CT scans were performed for diagnostic evaluation; 3D reconstructions are presented. Assessment of the stability of this fracture/luxation is difficult to assess, but due to the severity of the neurologic deficits, significant instability must be assumed. Provided adequate stability can be achieved with surgical intervention, the prognosis is good to excellent.

Options for Repair Methods

Segmental spinal stabilization is not a technique indicated in this size of patient. However, cross pins and methyl methacrylate cement should be considered. The technique is well reported and successful, but does require acrylic cement leading to an increased chance of infection. Plate fixation should also be considered. DCPs are a poor choice especially in this area. The plate must be pressed to the bone which is difficult in the lower thoracic area due to the rib heads. Disarticulating the ribs has been described, but is more invasive and painful. Locking plates, especially multi-planar contourable locking plates can be applied close to, but not directly on, the uneven contours of the vertebrae and provide stability.

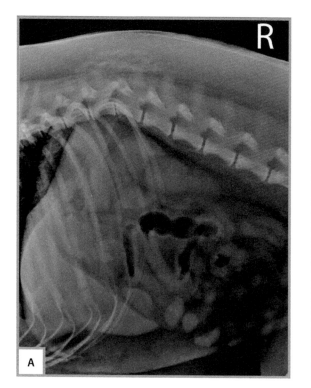

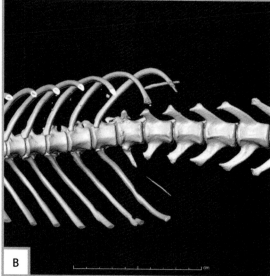

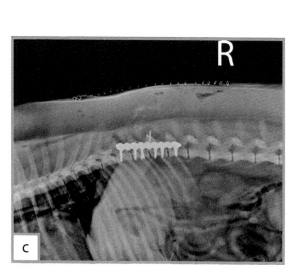

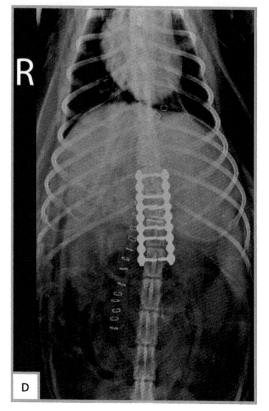

Figure 2.10 (A) Preoperative: lateral radiographic view; (B) Preoperative: ventrodorsal view of a 3D rendering from computed tomography (CT); (C) Postoperative: lateral view; (D) Postoperative: ventrodorsal view. *(Continued)*

Closed, Fracture/Luxation of the T12–13 Vertebrae *continued*

Surgery Report

Care was taken in transporting and positioning the patient under anesthesia. The patient was placed in the ventral recumbent position and an approach to the thoracolumbar vertebrae through a dorsal incision was performed from approximately T8 to L2. The area of luxation was identified and the luxation reduced using towel clamps placed on the T12 and T13 dorsal spinal processes. The more lateral cranial facets of T13 were pulled dorsally, and the narrower caudal facets of T12 were pushed ventrally until the T12/13 facet was anatomically reduced. When this reduction was maintained, two 1.1 mm (17 gauge) Kirschner wires were placed across the left and right facets from medial-to-lateral. Further elevation of hypaxial musculature was performed exposing the ventral aspect of the facels and rib heads. A 9-hole, 2.7 mm locking plate was contoured and positioned so that two screws would engage vertebrae T11 through L1 from the left side of the vertebrae. Two 2.7 mm cortical screws were placed into screw holes 3 and 4 and into the body of T12, and two screws were placed in screw holes 6 and 7 and into the body of T13. Further screws were placed into the body of T11 and L1. The same procedure was performed on the right side with the same plate and screw positioning. The vertebral luxation was manually checked for stability and the approach closed routinely.

Postoperative Evaluation of Fracture Repair (Figures 2.10C–D)

Criteria	Assessment	Details
Alignment	Optimal	The vertebral column has been anatomically reduced.
Apposition	Good	The disk space has been restored to near normal distance.
Apparatus	Good	Two plates were used. There are six screws cranial and caudal to the fracture/luxation. There are a total of four screws in T12 and T13. There are a total of two screws in T11 and L1. It would have been preferable to have four screws in T11 and L1, but the distances between holes in this plate did not allow this without screws entering disk spaces. The screws engage the body of the vertebrae and cross midline in most cases.

Follow-up at 10 Weeks (Figures 2.10E–F)

Criteria	Assessment
Alignment	Unchanged
Apposition	Unchanged
Apparatus	Unchanged
Activity	The cranial endplate of T13 appears to be healed with minimal callus. The goal of surgery was to stabilize the luxation with fibrous tissue to re-establish the stability of the vertebral motion units. Fusion of the spine was not the goal nor achieved. The vertebrae could still move as in a normal spine but they are constrained by the apparatus. Continued force on the moveable spine may be sufficient to impart enough force to fatigue the apparatus resulting in breakage of the screws and plates. In this case, if it resulted in pain, the apparatus would be removed. The patient was discharged with slow return to activity and weight loss. They were instructed to return in 6–12 months for follow-up radiographs.

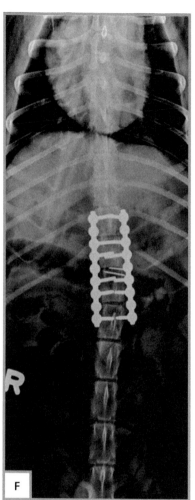

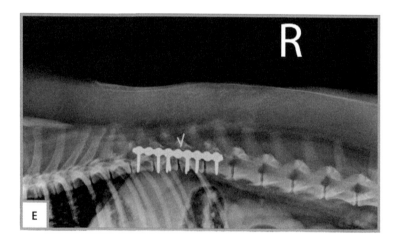

Figure 2.10 (Continued) (E) Follow-up at 10 Weeks: lateral view; (F) Follow-up at 10 Weeks: ventrodorsal view.

Closed, Left, Sacroiliac Luxation with a Fracture of the Sacral Wing

Signalment and History

A 4-year, 4-month-old, neutered, female miniature Dachshund, weighing 3.5 kg, was assumed to have been in a motor vehicle accident as she was found roadside by a neighbor. She was otherwise in good condition.

Patient Assessment

Radiographs revealed pelvic fractures, but thoracic and abdominal radiographs were within normal limits. Her bladder could be palpated and visualized radiographically. Neurologic examination revealed no abnormalities and the patient had sensation to the lateral digits of the caudal limbs, anus and tail; suggesting normal function of the sciatic, pudendal and caudal nerves. Even though radiographs were unremarkable, there was a possibility that the patient might have been run over, with resultant soft tissue trauma. This includes damage to and devitalization of skin in the pelvic area.

Fracture Assessment

Closed, left sacroiliac luxation with a fracture of the sacral wing, displaced cranially (Figures 2.11A–B). Sacroiliac luxations can be treated conservatively if they are stable, there is little compromise to diameter of the pelvic canal and proper orientation of the coxofemoral joint is maintained. Stability is assessed by direct palpation of the ilial wing; checking for motion, and observing if the patient is able to ambulate on that limb. Most sacroiliac luxations should be stabilized surgically. Sacroiliac luxations are often accompanied by fractures in segments of sacrum. If there is a very large segment of sacrum fractured, or if there is a sacral fracture, the prognosis is less good due to the potential for nerve damage. Surgical repair is much more difficult. If sacroiliac luxations are properly reduced, healing most often occurs without complication.

Options for Repair Methods

Pelvic-floor fractures of the pubis and ischium need not be surgically repaired. Attention is made to the weight-bearing segment, which in this case was compromised only at the sacroiliac joint. Lag screw fixation is the most common method of repair, and minimally invasive techniques have been described.[43] Fluoroscopy is used, when available, to assure proper screw placement. Other techniques such as external fixation have been described. The approach can be ventral or dorsal, though visualization of the sacrum is far superior with a dorsal approach. Single lag screws, double lag screws, or lag screw and Kirschner wire have been described. In soft bone, a washer or small plate is used to prevent the head of the screw from pulling through the wing of the ilium. It is essential to have the screw engage greater than 60 percent of the sacrum and not invade the vertebral canal or L7/S1 intervertebral foramen.

Surgery Report

The patient was placed in the right lateral recumbent position and effort was made to stop the patient leaning dorsally or ventrally. An approach to the wing of the ilium and dorsal aspect of the sacrum was performed. The wing of the ilium was displaced ventrally by carefully placing a Hohmann retractor on the ventral aspect of the wing of the sacrum and levering the ilium. The sacrum and surrounding structures were identified. The notch along the cranial border of the sacrum and the crescent-shaped auricular cartilage along the caudal-ventral aspect of the lateral sacrum are used as landmarks in locating the area for screw insertion into the sacral body; a target of about 1 cm diameter.

The landmark for drilling the hole in the sacrum was two-thirds the dorsal-to-ventral distance of the sacral wing, measured from the most dorsal aspect of the sacrum. The L7/S1 disk was probed to help with localization. There was a divot in the sacrum at this spot. Fibrous tissue was removed from this area to help with screw placement later. The direction of the drill was perpendicular to the floor with the

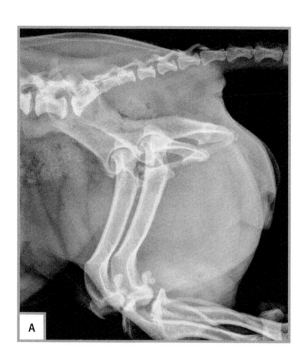

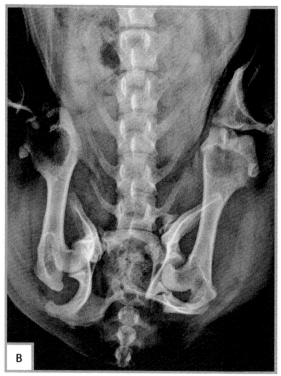

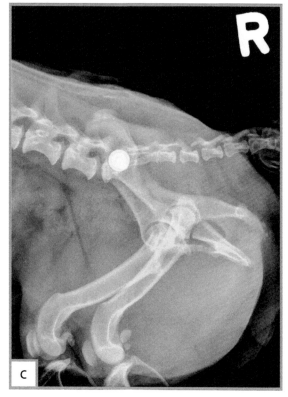

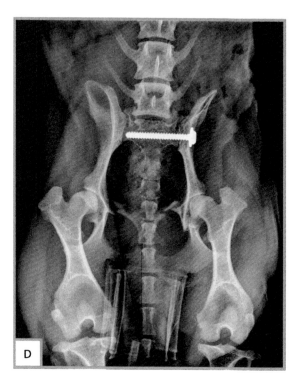

Figure 2.11 (A) Preoperative: lateral view; (B) Preoperative: ventrodorsal view; (C) Postoperative: lateral view; (D) Postoperative: ventrodorsal view.

(Continued)

Closed, Left, Sacroiliac Luxation with a Fracture of the Sacral Wing *continued*

patient positioned properly (as above), but this was not perpendicular to the flat surface of the sacrum. There is variability amongst patients such that the angle of the drill hole cannot be definitively described.[44] This problem was best solved by gentle palpation of the ventral aspect of the sacrum close to the midline for orientation. The sciatic nerve and branches of the internal iliac artery were in this position and care was taken to avoid damaging these structures.

A 2.0 mm drill bit was used to drill into the sacrum. The drill was removed and fluoroscopy was used to confirm proper screw placement. The depth of the hole was measured and compared to measurement from digital radiographs for the width of the sacrum plus one ilial wing. The sacral hole

was tapped. The Hohmann retractor was removed and the ilial wing palpated from the medial aspect to identify the small prominence that interdigitates with the divot of the sacrum. A 2.7 mm drill hole was drilled from the lateral aspect of the ilium to this prominence. The width of the ilial wing was measured and a 2.7 mm screw was selected, based on digital radiographs and measurements of the sacrum plus ilium. The 2.7 mm cortical screw with a washer was placed through the ilium. The ilium was retracted caudally using Kern bone-holding forceps so that the screw could be seen engaging the sacrum before tightening. As the screw was tightened, it could clearly be seen lagging the wing of the ilium to the sacrum and not displaced ventrally. The approach was closed routinely.

Postoperative Evaluation of Fracture Repair (Figures 2.11C–D)

Criteria	Assessment	Details
Alignment	Optimal	The ilial wing is at the proper position and the pelvic canal is re-established.
Apposition	Optimal	The sacroiliac joint space has been restored to near normal distance.
Apparatus	Optimal	The wing of the ilium is tightly lagged to the sacrum.

Follow-up at 8 Weeks (Figures 2.11E–F)

Criteria	Assessment
Alignment	Unchanged
Apposition	Unchanged
Apparatus	The screw had backed out approximately 1 mm.
Activity	The area of the luxation with fractured segment of sacrum appeared to have boney bridging. The patient was slowly returned to normal activity and the owner was informed that pain would likely ensue if the screw continued to migrate. Appropriate resolution would be screw removal.

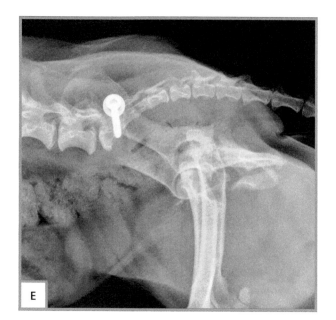
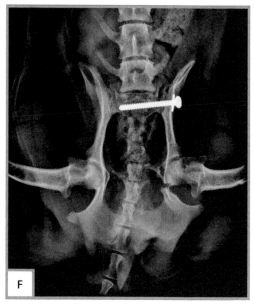

Figure 2.11 (Continued) (E) Follow-up at 8 Weeks: lateral view; (F) Follow-up at 8 Weeks: ventrodorsal view.

Closed, Right, Sacroiliac Luxation and Fracture of the Sacrum

Signalment and History
A 4-year-old, castrated, male Pomeranian weighing 10 kg was presented on referral following a motor vehicle accident. The patient had been administered pain medication and an antibiotic.

Patient Assessment
The patient was quiet, alert and responsive but non-ambulatory in the pelvic limbs and was painful on manipulation of pelvic structures. The body condition score was 8/9. There was sensation to the medial and lateral pelvic limbs digits, tail, and anus. Complete blood count and serum chemistries were within normal limits. Thoracic and abdominal radiographs did not reveal pulmonary contusions and the diaphragm was intact. The abdominal wall, bladder, and cranial pubic tendon could be visualized as normal. There was a laceration in the left inguinal area that was clipped and thoroughly lavaged followed by placement of a wet-to-dry bandage. Despite his stable condition, the patient sustained severe trauma and could have been run over by the vehicle.

Fracture Assessment
Closed, right sacroiliac luxation and fracture of the cranial wing of the sacrum displaced cranially 2 cm. Closed, long oblique fracture of the left ilial shaft, ventrally displaced and overriding 2 cm. Multiple fractures of the pelvic floor were present (Figures 2.12A–B).

Pelvic fractures are assessed with attention to the weight-bearing segments that include the femoral head, coxofemoral joint, acetabulum, ilium, sacroiliac joint, and sacrum. Fractures or luxations of these structures should be surgically repaired. This patient was likely run over by a vehicle, giving rise to multiple pelvic fractures. When this occurs there is considerable soft tissue damage in addition to pelvic fractures. Attention should be given to assessment of the abdominal wall and bladder. If compromise to the bladder or urinary tract is suspected, then abdominocentesis should be performed followed by comparison of the aspirated fluid to peripheral serum creatinine. If abdominal fluid creatinine is higher, then a contrast cystourethrogram should be performed. In the event that a compromised bladder is diagnosed, it should be repaired once the patient is metabolically stable.

In addition to the bladder, patient neurologic function must be assessed. There was a right ischial shaft fracture sustained by this patient, prompting assessment of the sciatic nerve which transits this area. Sensation to the lateral pelvic digits that are supplied by the sciatic nerve is used to assess the sciatic nerve. In addition, sensation to the tail and anus must be assessed in pelvic trauma that includes sacral fracture(s).

When patients sustain pelvic fractures from a motor vehicle accident, integrity of the pelvic skin must be assessed. This is especially true for obese patients as the skin can get pulled away from underlying soft tissues and subsequently become devitalized. Accurately assessing viability of skin immediately following injury can be difficult as it may seem pliable and only somewhat cool. A period of 24–72 hours may be necessary for skin to demonstrate signs of devitalization; cold to the touch, hard and discolored. Still, the owner must be made aware of this potential complication. If the skin becomes devitalized, it must be surgically debrided and the wound closed or left open to heal by second intention.

Options for Repair Methods
Left ilial shaft fracture: This is a long oblique fracture and lag screw fixation has been described. However, due to the width of the ilium and limited bone stock for screw purchase, this may be technically difficult. Cerclage wiring can be attempted, but often proves insufficiently stable. Plate fixation is commonly used in ilial shaft fractures and DCPs or locking plates may be used. Locking screws are often used in thin bone such as the ilium because the holding power is greater in most situations.

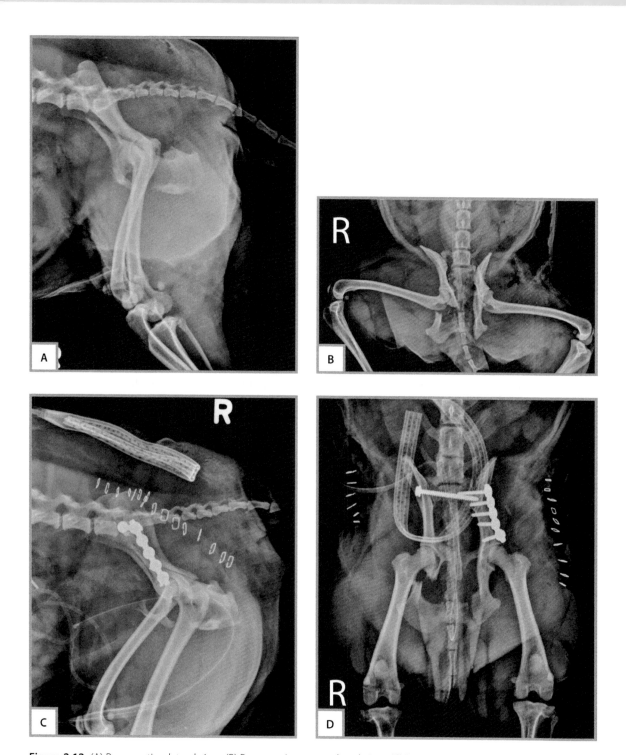

Figure 2.12 (A) Preoperative: lateral view; (B) Preoperative: ventrodorsal view; (C) Postoperative: lateral view; (D) Postoperative: ventrodorsal view.

(Continued)

Closed, Right, Sacroiliac Luxation and Fracture of the Sacrum *continued*

Right sacroiliac luxation: Sacroiliac luxations are often repaired by the lag screw technique. A consideration for this patient is that his right-sided luxation is accompanied by a concurrent sacral fracture. Sacral fractures can dramatically complicate sacroiliac luxations. Sacral fractures alone are difficult because lag screw fixation leads to collapse of the fracture and medial displacement of the hemi-pelvis when the fracture is compressed. Sacral nerve roots can become entrapped leading to pain and dysfunction from the pelvic and pudendal nerves. In many sacroiliac luxation cases a part of the sacrum, usually the sacral wing (ala), is fractured. Lag screwing the ilium to the flat surface of the sacral articulation will usually lateralize the hemi-pelvis and acetabulum to a normal anatomic position. If the sacrum is fractured, lateralization may not occur or be incomplete. The degree of this complication depends on the size and configuration of the sacral fracture.

Surgery Report

The patient was first placed in the right lateral recumbent position and an approach to the ilium through a lateral incision was performed. The ilial fracture was reduced and held in compression with Kern bone-holding forceps. A 5-hole 2.7 mm locking plate was contoured to the ventral lateral surface of the ilium. The plate was applied by placing screws in holes 4 and 5 first, followed by screws in holes 1–3, in sequence. The incision was closed routinely.

The patient was thereafter placed in the left lateral recumbent position and an approach to the wing of the ilium and dorsal aspect of the sacrum was performed. The wing of the ilium was displaced ventrally to expose the sacroiliac joint and fracture of the sacrum. The notch along the cranial border of the sacrum and the crescent-shaped auricular cartilage along the caudal-ventral aspect of the lateral sacrum are used as landmarks in locating the area for screw insertion into the sacral body; a target of about 1 cm diameter. Some of these landmarks were estimated due to the presence of the sacral fracture. The ventral aspect of the sacral body was carefully probed with a hemostat as an aid for drilling into the sacral body. A 2.0 mm drill bit was used to drill across the sacral body and into the ilial wing on the contralateral (left) side. A 2.5 mm drill bit was then used to over-drill this hole. The order in which these tasks were performed was so that the 2.0 mm drill hole could be redirected if needed without compromise of too much bone. The drill-hole depth was measured. A location on the ilial wing corresponding to the center of the sacrum was estimated by palpation of the sacroiliac joint and fragment of the sacrum, through which a 3.5 mm glide hole was drilled. The depth of this hole was measured. A 3.5 mm screw with washer, the approximate combined length of the sacrum plus ilium, was selected and placed through the wing of the ilium so as to protrude through the medial aspect several millimeters. The tip of the screw was then directed into the sacral hole and visually seen to penetrate the sacral screw-hole. The screw was tightened and lagging of the ilium to the sacrum was confirmed by palpation of the two compressing segments during tightening of the screw.

It was noted during both approaches that there was avulsion of the skin from deeper tissues resulting in a large area of dead space. The skin continued to appear viable at that time. A large, closed-suction drain was placed into this pocket and suction was applied for 5 days. The skin remained viable.

Postoperative Evaluation of Fracture Repair (Figures 2.12C–D)

Left Ilial Shaft Fracture

Criteria	Assessment	Details
Alignment	Optimal	The fracture is anatomically reduced.
Apposition	Good	A fracture line can still be seen caudally.
Apparatus	Sufficient	Only two locking screws engage the caudal ilial segment and only three engage the cranial segment. More screw purchase would be desirable. However, the caudal bone segment does not appear to allow more screw purchase.

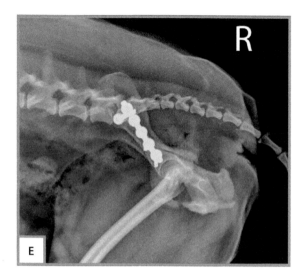

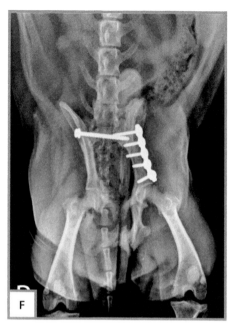

Figure 2.12 (Continued) (E) Follow-up at 8 Weeks: lateral view; (F) Follow-up at 8 Weeks: ventrodorsal view.

Right Sacroiliac Luxation

Criteria	Assessment	Details
Alignment	Sufficient	The hemi-pelvis is medially displaced resulting in medial displacement of the right acetabulum by approximately 1 cm. The orientation of the acetabulum is still adequate and the pelvic canal is substantively maintained.
Apposition	Good	The fracture luxation is compressed.
Apparatus	Sufficient	The lag screw spans the entire sacrum and is therefore of Sufficient length. The screw is centered in the body of the sacrum.

Follow-up at 8 Weeks (Figures 2.12E–F)

Left Ilial Shaft Fracture

Criteria	Assessment
Alignment	Unchanged
Apposition	Unchanged
Apparatus	Unchanged
Activity	The fracture appears healed ventrally and medially, but a fracture line is still visible dorsally over the acetabulum.

Right Sacroiliac Luxation

Criteria	Assessment
Alignment	The medial displacement of the right acetabulum appears to have increased by approximately 5 mm compared to postoperative images.
Apposition	Unchanged
Apparatus	Unchanged
Activity	The sacral fracture appears healed. In addition, there appears to be signs of early osteoarthritis in the right coxofemoral joint. The patient was ambulating well but with some gait abnormality of the right pelvic limb, yet was allowed to slowly return to normal activity and was continued on a weight-reduction program.

Closed, Long Oblique Fracture of the Left Ilial Shaft

Signalment and History
A 6-year-old, intact, female Chihuahua, weighing 4.1 kg sustained multiple pelvic fractures from a motor vehicle accident.

Patient Assessment
Considering multiple pelvic fractures, soft tissue and neurologic damage are a potential concern and should be assessed. There are often injuries in addition to orthopedic, which can be life threatening. In addition, soft tissue and skin can be damaged and can be, or soon become devitalized. In this case soft tissues were not severely damaged and neurologic function was intact. Given pelvic fractures in an intact female, owners should be counseled that future pregnancies could have complications and neutering should be considered after fracture recovery.

Fracture Assessment
Closed, long oblique left ilial shaft fracture, displaced ventrally and overriding 1 cm. Closed right sacroiliac luxation, displaced ventrally and over-riding 2 cm (Figures 2.13A–B). In assessing pelvic fractures, fixation is usually limited to the weight-bearing segment. This includes the femoral neck and head, acetabulum, ilial shaft, sacroiliac joint, and sacrum. Although most patients have fractures of other pelvic structures, these are generally not considered weight-bearing and are not repaired. This patient also has bilateral ischial fractures. These are painful and there is potential for sciatic nerve damage or incorporation of the sciatic nerve into the healing fracture callus. These fractures are usually treated conservatively.

The sacroiliac luxation is considerably displaced and unstable. The segment of right hemipelvis is displaced into the pelvic canal. This could cause an abnormal gait and compromise to the pelvic canal. Surgical correction is recommended in these cases for faster ambulation, correction of pelvic conformation, and Optimal gait.

Options for Repair Methods
Ilial shaft fractures are commonly repaired with plate fixation. Although DCPs are commonly used, locking plate systems can also be used; arguably they provide an advantage given the thin bone of the ilial wing. Lag-screw fixation has been described for long oblique fractures of the shaft of the ilium but they present challenges in smaller breeds of dogs. Sacroiliac luxations are most frequently repaired with lag screw fixation.

Surgery Report
The patient was placed in the right lateral recumbent position. An approach to the ilium through a lateral incision was performed. A 2.0 mm 8-hole DCP plate was contoured to the general shape of the ilium and applied to the fracture, although there was some medial deviation of the caudal segment. Two 2.0 mm screws were first placed in screw holes 6 and 7. Thereafter, the cranial plate was manually pressed to the wing of the ilium; thereby lateralizing the caudal aspect of the ilium. Screws 3 and 4 were applied in dynamic compression. The remaining screws were applied in the order 5–8–1–2. All screws were selected for lengths to only engage the ilium and not the sacrum. Routine closure was performed.

The patient was then positioned in the left lateral recumbent position. An approach to the wing of the ilium and dorsal aspect of the sacrum was performed. In these fractures, the ilium is usually displaced craniodorsally, therefore the wing of the ilium was forced ventrally to expose the crescent-shaped cartilage of the lateral sacrum. Utilizing the notch along the cranial border of the sacrum and the crescent-shaped articular cartilage of the lateral sacrum as landmarks, the target for screw placement into the sacrum was identified. (The sacral tap hole should be drilled just caudal to this notch and just cranial to the crescent-shaped articular cartilage.) A 2.0 mm hole was drilled and tapped at this target. (Viewing the lateral surface of

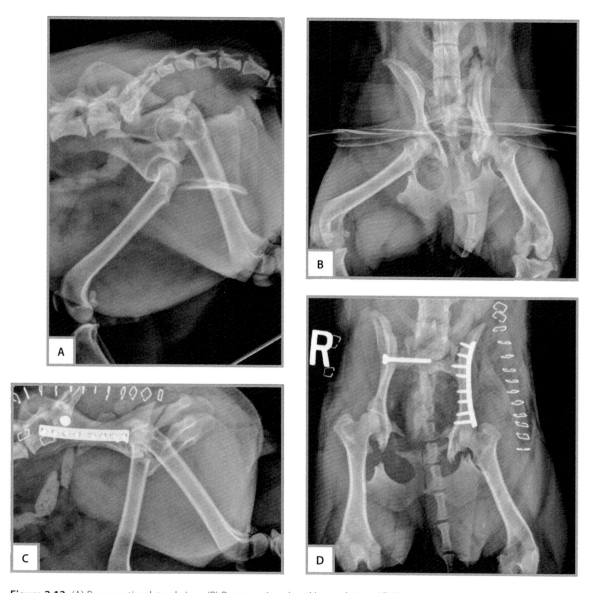

Figure 2.13 (A) Preoperative: lateral view; (B) Preoperative: dorsal/ventral view; (C) Postoperative: lateral view; (D) Postoperative: dorsal/ventral view.

(Continued)

Closed, Long Oblique Fracture of the Left Ilial Shaft *continued*

the ilium, target for screw placement is determined by first visually dividing the length of the straight portion of the dorsal iliac crest into two equal parts. The cranial/caudal location of the target hole lies in the center of the caudal half, while the dorsal/ventral location lies in the center of that half. Target accuracy can be confirmed by palpation of the roughened articular surface of the medial ilium.) A 2.7 mm hole was made in the ilium and the depth of the ilial hole was measured. A screw with the additive length of the ilial hole and sacral hole was introduced through the ilial glide hole and into the sacral hole, thereby compressing the ilium to the sacrum in a lag fashion. Routine closure was performed.

Postoperative Evaluation of Fracture Repair (Figures 2.13C–D)

Left Ilial Shaft Fracture

Criteria	Assessment	Details
Alignment	Optimal	The fracture is reduced and has re-established the normal contour of the pelvis on this side.
Apposition	Good	The fracture line is still visible, but compression appears to have been achieved.
Apparatus	Good	There are four screws on each side of the fracture, each engaging two cortices. The bone is thin and the thread profile of 2.0 mm screws is fine, making screw pullout a concern. This is an older patient and likely had good ilial bone integrity. Locking screw systems or doubling locking screw plates may have been a better choice. Screw 3 appears to engage the sacrum. With motion at the sacroiliac joint, a single screw may be subject to back out, breakage, cause bone lysis, or pain. If the sacrum is to be engaged, then more than one screw should engage the sacrum as much as possible.

Right Sacroiliac Luxation

Criteria	Assessment	Details
Alignment	Optimal	The luxation has been anatomically reduced and the hemipelvis has been lateralized such that configuration of the pelvic canal is restored to near normal.
Apposition	Sufficient	The sacroiliac luxation has been reduced and compressed. The amount of contact apposition is minimal and suggests potential for instability.
Apparatus	Good	The 2.7 mm screw appears to engage nearly 60 percent the width of the sacrum. Placement of the lag screw appears to be in the center of the sacral target. Adding an additional screw could have been considered, although the sacral target zone is small. Adding a Kirschner wire could be considered, but the additional strength provided by a small wire in this patient would be unlikely to add much to the mechanical stability of the fixation.

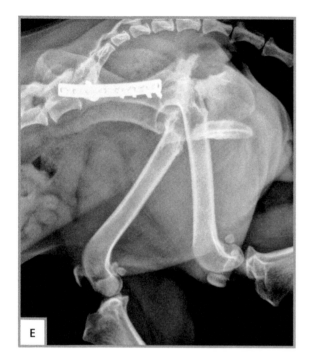
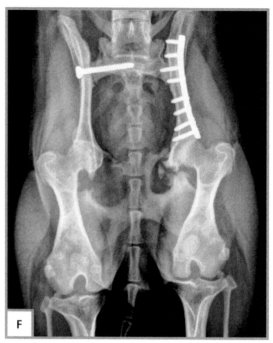

Figure 2.13 (Continued) (E) Follow-up at 7 Weeks: lateral view; (F) Follow-up at 7 Weeks: dorsal/ventral view.

Follow-up at 7 Weeks (Figures 2.13E–F)

Left Ilial Shaft Fracture

Criteria	Assessment
Alignment	Unchanged
Apposition	Unchanged
Apparatus	Unchanged
Activity	There is minimal callus formation and the fracture lines are only barely visible. There is bridging activity at the pubis and ishium, however, boney union has not been achieved.

Right Sacroiliac Luxation

Criteria	Assessment
Alignment	Unchanged
Apposition	Unchanged
Apparatus	Unchanged
Activity	There is radiographic evidence of boney activity at the sacroiliac joint and this joint has not fused.

Closed, Short Oblique Fracture of the Right Ilial Shaft

Signalment and History
A 2.5-year-old, neutered, female Lassapoo, weighing 6 kg was presented with trauma to the pelvis after falling from a height of approximately one meter.

Patient Assessment
The patient was in good condition, but was non-ambulatory on the right pelvic limb. There was no other apparent trauma. The patient could ambulate on the other three limbs. Neurologic examination, including perineal reflex, was within normal limits. There was pain sensation to the right lateral pelvic limb demonstrating sensory function to the right sciatic nerve. The fracture could be palpated on rectal examination and was noted to invade the pelvic canal. Thoracic and abdominal radiographs were recommended, but not performed on request of the owner.

Fracture Assessment
Closed, short oblique fracture of the right ilial shaft, 1 cm cranial to the acetabulum, displaced medially and over-riding 2 cm (Figures 2.14A–B). This is a relatively low-energy fracture in an area of good blood supply. Given proper stabilization, this fracture would have a good prognosis for healing.

Options for Repair Methods
Conservative treatment would not be recommended, as the fracture was in the weight-bearing segment and the pelvic canal was compromised. Plating would be the preferred method of fixation. Either locking or non-locking plates could be selected. Dynamic compression plating should provide compression across the fracture line. The ilium is thin in this sized patient and screw-holding strength would be low. There is a small amount of bone in the distal bone segment, constraining the number of cortices for screw engagement. Locking plates would have the advantage of better holding power in this segment of bone. In addition, some locking plates such as the String of Pearls (SOP) system can be nested to increase the number of screws engaging a small segment of bone, thereby increasing the construct's AMI.

Surgery Report
The patient was placed in the left lateral recumbent position rather than through the ilium through a lateral incision was performed. The perimysium of the gluteal muscles was incised giving access to the ventral lateral border of the ilium. The gluteals were elevated and retracted with an Army/Navy retractor. The fracture line was debrided and the caudal fracture fragment was grasped with Kern bone-holding forceps. The fracture was reduced, excepting minor medial-displacement of the caudal pelvic fragment. A 5-hole, 2.7 mm SOP plate was contoured to the dorsal-lateral aspect of the ilium and over the acetabulum. The plate was then over contoured to duplicate the shape of the contra lateral, intact ilium. The plate was applied to the caudal bone segment first with two 2.7 mm screws. The cranial aspect of the plate was then 'pushed' flush to the ilial wing, thereby lateralizing the caudal hemipelvis. Three 2.7 mm screws were placed in the ilial wing. A second 2.7 mm 4-hole SOP plate was contoured and twisted to lie ventral to the first plate. Three screws were placed for fixation in the 4-hole plate; two screws in the proximal bone segment and one screw in the distal bone segment. Screw hole 3 of this plate overlays the fracture line and was left empty. Closure was routine.

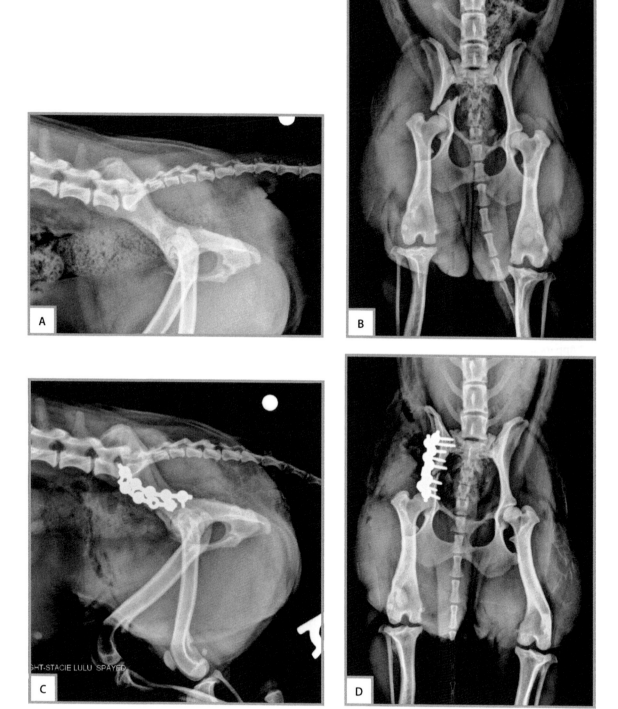

Figure 2.14 (A) Preoperative: lateral view; (B) Preoperative: ventral/dorsal view; (C) Postoperative: lateral view; (D) Postoperative: ventral/dorsal view.

(Continued)

Closed, Short Oblique Fracture of the Right Ilial Shaft *continued*

Postoperative Evaluation of Fracture Repair (Figures 2.14C–D)

Criteria	Assessment	Details
Alignment	Optimal	Anatomic conformation of the pelvis was re-established.
Apposition	Good	The fracture line on the medial aspect of the ilial shaft is seen, suggesting over-reduction or lack of compression at the fracture line.
Apparatus	Good	Nesting of the SOP plates will allow Good stabilization of the fracture. The caudal bone segment would only allow three total screws; however, they are positioned so that they will support each other in bending and torsion. The screws engaged only the ilium and did not engage the sacroiliac joint. Engaging the sacroiliac joint can lead to pain or screw loosening unless the fixation fully stabilizes the joint.

Follow-up at 9 Weeks (Figures 2.14E–F)

Criteria	Assessment
Alignment	Unchanged
Apposition	Unchanged
Apparatus	Unchanged
Activity	There is bridging callus across the fracture line though the fracture line can still be visualized radiographically. There is mild subluxation of the coxofemoral joint. The patient was slowly returned to normal activity.

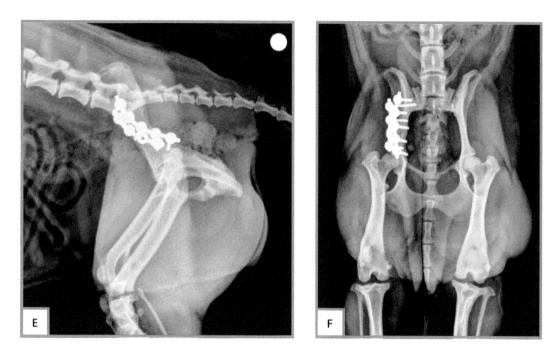

Figure 2.14 (Continued) (E) Follow-up at 9 Weeks: lateral view; (F) Follow-up at 9 Weeks: ventral/dorsal view.

Closed, Comminuted Fracture of the Left Ilium and Central Acetabulum

Signalment and History
A 7-year-old, neutered, female Labrador Retriever weighing 28 kg sustained skull and pelvic trauma from a motor vehicle accident. This report details the pelvic fractures only. The patient presented in distributive shock.

Patient Assessment
Thoracic radiographs demonstrated pneumothorax with rib fractures, pulmonary contusion, and multiple skull fractures. Abdominal radiographs demonstrated lumbar streaking suggestive of extra-peritoneal hemorrhage. The patient was depressed, but was able to be aroused and had direct and consensual pupillary eye reflexes. A full neurologic examination was to be performed following resuscitation. The patient was placed on IV fluids with full shock doses administered as repeated assessments dictated. Pulse oximetery was monitored together with respirations and mentation. Repeated thoracic radiographs were performed three hours after admission. The patient responded well to initial treatment. A neurologic examination revealed normal mentation and cranial nerve examination gave no suggestion of increased intracranial pressure or brain damage.

A thorough discussion of polytrauma issues is not within the scope of this text. However, the extent of trauma to the patient must be assessed. Total patient assessment is important for polytrauma cases due to the high risk for complications including infection and delayed bone healing. The patient should be thoroughly stabilized metabolically prior to fracture fixation, wherein a period of 2–3 days is not considered excessive.

Fracture Assessment
Closed comminuted fracture of the shaft of the left ilium and central acetabulum, displaced cranially 1 cm (Figures 2.15A–B). Unlike most pelvic fractures, the contralateral os coxae was not fractured.

Acetabular fractures can be identified principally as cranial, central, caudal, or comminuted. Caudal fractures can, in some situations, be treated conservatively; provided the caudal articulating fracture segment is small. Comminuted fractures can be difficult to manage and in some situations, require a femoral head and neck ostectomy. Cranial and central acetabular fractures, as well as ilial shaft fractures, should be repaired with open reduction and internal fixation to ensure excellent apposition of the articular surface, and because these are associated with weight-bearing of the joint. Interfragmentary compression should be performed whenever possible.

Options for Repair Methods
These fractures involve both the acetabulum and ilial shaft so fixation techniques that span both fractures should be considered. Dynamic compression is most often chosen, but buttress fixation is an option if compression cannot be achieved. In this case, the degree of comminution of the ilium would make reduction of the fracture fragments challenging, and compression especially difficult. Alternatively, buttress fixation with a locking plate system could include the major bone fragments. Likely, more than one fixation device would be needed. DCPs placed in buttress, neutral, or perhaps load fashion and crossing some of the fracture lines may also be appropriate, depending on constraints observed intraoperatively.

Surgery Report
The patient was placed in the right lateral recumbent position and a combined craniodorsal and caudodorsal approach to the hip, via osteotomy of the greater trochanter, was performed in routine fashion. Prior to osteotomy of the greater trochanter, a 1.5 mm drill bit was used to create both the Steinmann pin tracks and a tunnel for passage of orthopedic wire anticipated with the

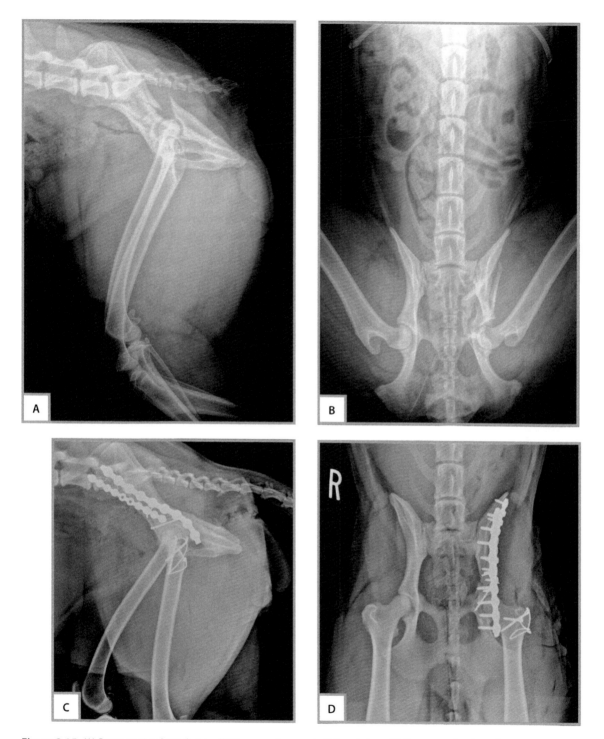

Figure 2.15 (A) Preoperative: lateral view; (B) Preoperative: ventral/dorsal view; (C) Postoperative: lateral view; (D) Postoperative: ventral/dorsal view.

(Continued)

tension band repair. The trochanteric osteotomy was performed with a sagittal saw. Visualization was maintained with Glepi and Army/Navy retractors. Intraoperatively, the craniodorsal joint capsule was observed to be torn and a cranial-to-central acetabular fracture was confirmed. Pointed reduction forceps were placed on the femoral neck and used to reduce the acetabular fracture. An additional pointed reduction forcep was used to reduce the long oblique fracture of the ilial shaft. A 1.6 mm (14 gauge) interfragmentary Kirschner wire was placed across the ilium and ischium just cranial to the acetabulum, beginning at the origin of the rectus femoris muscle and directed dorsally and caudally to the ischiatic spine. A second 1.6 mm interfragmentary Kirschner wire was placed across the ilial shaft fracture, starting from the origin of the rectus femoris muscle and directed dorsally

and cranially. A 9 hole 3.5 mm locking plate was contoured and placed from the cranial ilial wing, dorsal to the acetabulum, coursing to the level of the ischiatic spine. Three screws engaged the ischium, three engaged the caudal ilial shaft and three engaged the ilial wing. Thereafter, a 10-hole 2.7 mm locking plate was contoured and placed from the ilial wing to the ilial shaft spanning the ilial shaft fracture line. Eight screws were placed in screw holes 1–4, and 7–10, leaving screw holes 5 and 6 open as they were over fracture lines.

The trochanteric osteotomy was reduced and 2.0 mm Steinmann pins were driven into the two preplaced holes. A 1.2 mm (16 gauge) tension band wire was placed in a figure-of-eight and twisted tight to complete the tension band. The approach was closed routinely.

Postoperative Evaluation of Fracture Repair (Figures 2.15C–D)

Criteria	Assessment	Details
Alignment	Good	The fracture is well aligned. Acetabular orientation is accurate with adequate dorsal acetabular coverage. This may be over represented in this radiograph due to positioning
Apposition	Acetabulum–Optimal	The acetabulum is anatomically reduced. Fracture lines of the ilium remain visible, especially in the ventral to dorsal view. The greater trochanter has been anatomically reduced.
Apparatus	Good	The locking plates include at least three screws in all bone segments, which are additionally supported by the Kirschner wires. Though the wires do not contribute to fragmentary compression, they do contribute to opposing shear forces at the fractures, the most critical being the acetabular fracture line. Addition of the second plate considerably increases the AMI of the construct. Multiple screws have purchase in the thin bone of the ilial wing. Screws to not cross the sacroiliac joint, and the tension band is of appropriately sized wire. In contrast to this case, two twists are described to allow optimal compression of the osteotomy tension band, as tightening with only one twist requires the orthopedic wire to slide around the Steinmann pins.

First Follow-up at 6 Weeks (Figures 2.15E–F)

Criteria	Assessment
Alignment	Unchanged
Apposition	Unchanged
Apparatus	Unchanged
Activity	There is mild callus formation on the medial aspect of the ilial fractures only, suggesting Good stability. Fracture lines are still noticeable at the ilial fractures suggesting incomplete healing.

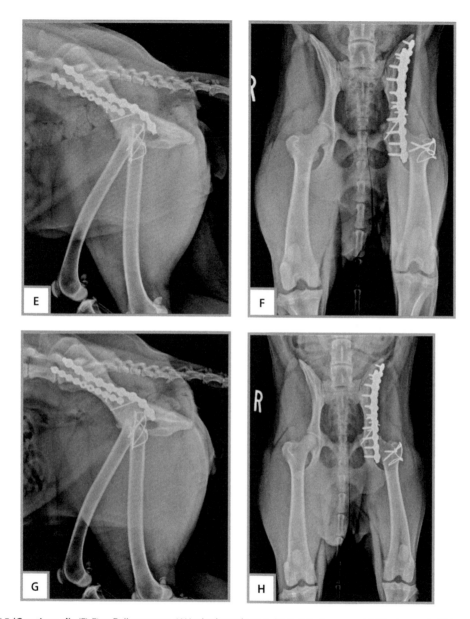

Figure 2.15 (Continued) (E) First Follow-up at 6 Weeks: lateral view; (F) First Follow-up at 6 Weeks: ventral/dorsal view; (G) Final Follow-up at 9 Weeks: lateral view; (H) Final Follow-up at 9 Weeks: ventral/dorsal view.

Final Follow-up at 9 Weeks (Figures 2.15G–H)

Criteria	Assessment
Alignment	Unchanged
Apposition	Unchanged
Apparatus	Unchanged
Activity	The callus has reduced in size and remodeled. Fracture lines are not apparent. There is mild-to-moderate osteoarthritis of the coxofemoral joint. The patient was returned to normal activity with instructions that pain and lameness could result from the osteoarthritis and medical management would be appropriate.

Closed, Bilateral, Central Acetabular Fractures

Signalment and History
A 6-month-old, neutered, female Labrador Retriever weighing 22 kg sustained pelvic trauma from being crushed by falling concrete blocks. The patient was acutely treated for pain and referred to the surgical hospital.

Patient Assessment
Thoracic and abdominal radiographs were within normal limits. Neurologic examination was within normal limits and sciatic nerve function was intact bilaterally. Although a young dog with very good healing potential, these are articular fractures in a growing dog and subsequent joint incongruity or direct cartilage damage to the joint may lead to osteoarthritis.

Fracture Assessment
Closed, bilateral, central acetabular fractures displaced ventrally and over-riding 1 cm (Figures 2.16A–B). Acetabular fractures can be cranial, central, caudal, or comminuted. Caudal fractures can, in some situations, be treated conservatively; provided the articulating fracture segment is small. Comminuted fractures can be difficult to manage and in some situations, require a femoral head and neck ostectomy. Cranial and central acetabular fractures should be repaired with open reduction and internal fixation to ensure excellent apposition of the articular surface.

Options for Repair Methods
Plate fixation is usually chosen for acetabular fractures, as this allows rigid fixation and compression at the fracture line. Either locking or DCPs can be used; though the later will allow interfragmentary compression. A variety of plates can be used depending on the fracture configuration. Offerings include specialized acetabular plates and highly contourable plates for ease of contouring. Acetabular bone in this patient will be soft and the security of screws anchoring a plate will be low. Locking plates may have superior benefit, as they may have lesser chance for disruption of fracture reduction upon screw tightening if the plate is not precisely contoured. Additionally, locking plates offer greater resistance to screw pull out.

Surgery Report
The patient was placed in the left lateral recumbent position and an approach to the craniodorsal and caudodorsal aspects of the right hip joint by osteotomy of the greater trochanter was performed. The fracture was reduced and held in reduction and compression with pointed reduction forceps. Small drill holes into the cortical bone were made to assist with forcep placement. A 4-hole 2.0 mm locking plate was contoured and placed along the dorsal acetabulum with four 2.0 mm screws. A second, 5-hole 2.0 mm was contoured and placed ventrally along the acetabular rim, leaving the center screw hole empty to avoid the fracture line. The greater trochanter was reduced and repaired with a tension band of 1.6 mm (14 gauge) Kirschner wires and 1 mm cerclage wire. The incision was closed routinely. The contralateral acetabular fracture was repaired in a like manner.

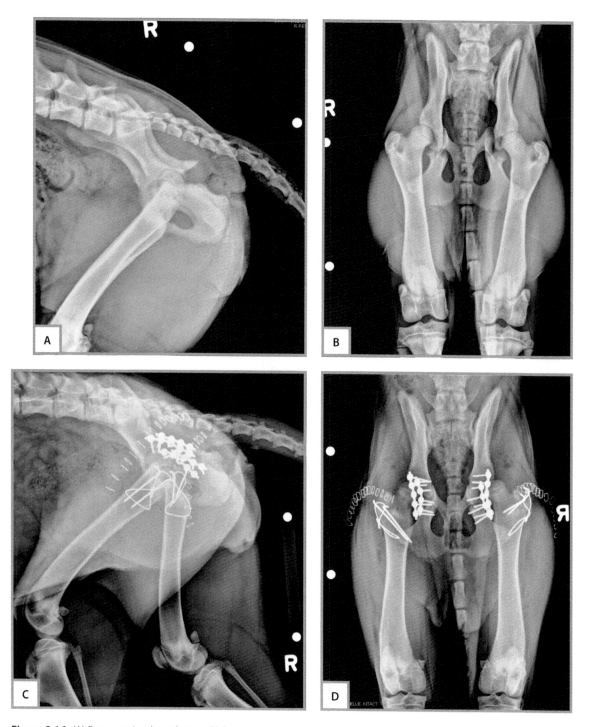

Figure 2.16 (A) Preoperative: lateral view; (B) Preoperative: ventral/dorsal view; (C) Postoperative: lateral view; (D) Postoperative: ventral/dorsal view.

(Continued)

Closed, Bilateral, Central Acetabular Fractures *continued*

Postoperative Evaluation of Fracture Repair (Figures 2.16C–D)

Criteria	Assessment	Details
Alignment	Optimal	The fractures are anatomically reduced.
Apposition	Good	The fracture lines can be seen on postoperative radiographs; but they are small. There is moderate subluxation of the coxofemoral joints.
Apparatus		2.0 mm plates and screws are small for this size patient. However, two plates would act together to greatly enhance the AMI of the fixation. The use of two smaller plates allowed the application of four screws per fracture segment. In softer juvenile bone this would have an advantage in screw-holding strength. A locking plate was used with angle-stable screws. Though small, the screws do not rely on thread-holding power and provide additional benefit in soft bone. Both tension bands were adequately placed. Two twists on the cerclage wire are preferred so as to more evenly distribute the applied tension.

Follow-up at 6 Weeks (Figures 2.16E–F)

Criteria	Assessment
Alignment	Unchanged
Apposition	Unchanged
Apparatus	Unchanged
Activity	Fractures have healed with moderate callus. There is moderate subluxation of the coxofemoral joints. The patient was slowly returned to normal activity and monitored for signs of coxofemoral joint osteoarthritis.

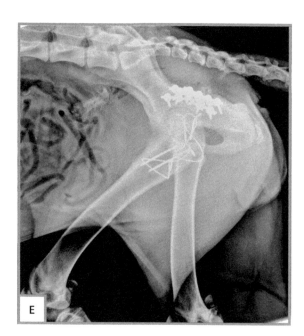

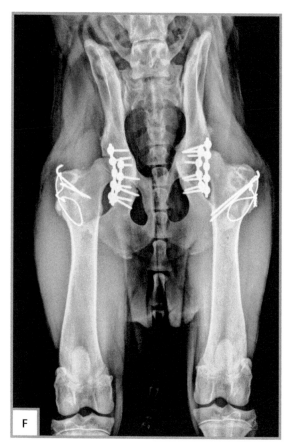

Figure 2.16 (Continued) (E) Follow-up at 6 Weeks: lateral view; (F) Follow-up at 6 Weeks: ventral/dorsal view.

Closed, Salter I Fracture of the Right Femoral Capital Physis

Signalment and History
An 8-month-old, neutered, female Neopolitan Mastiff weighing 37 kg sustained a coxofemoral joint fracture from falling on a slippery surface four days prior to presentation.

Patient Assessment
This is a large, but young patient with good healing potential. At this age there is some, but little more, skeletal growth anticipated. These fractures should be operated as soon as possible because continued movement of the hip will damage the physis and compromise blood supply to the femoral head and neck.

Fracture Assessment
Closed Salter I fracture of the right femoral capital physis (Figures 2.17A–B).

Options for Repair Methods
Techniques described include divergent Kirschner wire fixation or lag screw fixation. Divergent Kirschner wires are somewhat difficult to place, but (in theory) can spare continued growth of the physis. Lag screw fixation is technically less difficult, but provides little purchase of the capital epiphysis, and yields a high probability for closing the physeal growth plate. A partially-threaded lag screw would be preferred, but a cortical screw placed in lag fashion would be adequate.

Surgery Report
An approach to the craniodorsal aspect of the right hip joint through a craniolateral incision was performed. An incision into the joint capsule was made with a No.15 blade and minimal periosteal elevation was performed to limit compromise to the local blood supply. Meyerding retractors allowed visualization of the fracture site. The fracture was reduced manually by internally rotating the hip and pushing the neck caudally to visualize proper reduction. The fracture was then again luxated. Using a 4.5 mm drill bit, a hole was drilled from the third trochanter to the middle of the physis, and the depth of this hole was measured. A drill guide with an outer diameter of 4.5 mm and inner diameter of 3.2 mm was place into this hole from the third trochanter. The fracture was then again reduced and a hole was drilled through the femoral capitis. The depth of this hole was measured, and a 4.5 mm screw was chosen from the depth of the hole in the femoral neck and the width of the capitus as measured from digital radiographs. The depth of the entire measured hole was considered, and the length of screw chosen would need to be less than this distance. The hole in the capitis was tapped and the screw inserted. The hip was then cycled through a range of motion; checking for crepitation that might suggest excessive screw length and joint invasion.

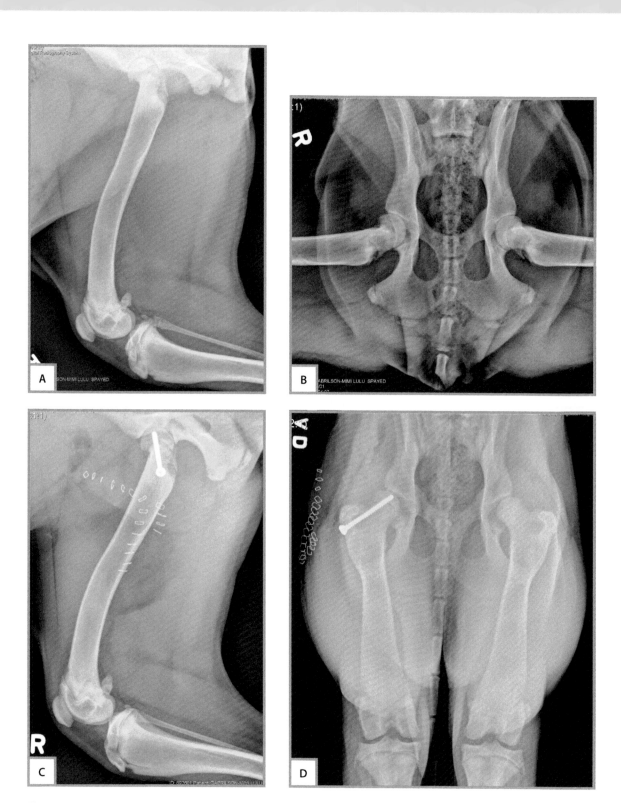

Figure 2.17 (A) Preoperative: lateral view; (B) Preoperative: dorsal/ventral view; (C) Postoperative: lateral view; (D) Postoperative: dorsal/ventral view.

(Continued)

Closed, Salter I Fracture of the Right Femoral Capital Physis *continued*

Postoperative Evaluation of Fracture Repair (Figures 2.17C–D)

Criteria	Assessment	Details
Alignment	Good	There is slight (2 mm) displacement of the capital physis.
Apposition	Optimal	The capital physis is compressed with a minimal fracture gap noted.
Apparatus	Optimal	The lag screw is placed correctly and engages the capital physis with four full threads engaging the capital epiphysis. A 4.5 mm screw has a pitch of 1.75 mm: therefore, 7 mm of 'bone' was purchased with the screw.

Follow-up at 4 Weeks (Figures 2.17E–F)

Criteria	Assessment
Alignment	Unchanged
Apposition	Unchanged
Apparatus	Unchanged
Activity	The fracture appears to have healed, with the physeal line no longer visible. There has been minimal callus formation, which is desirable for this type of fracture close to a joint. The hip appears somewhat subluxated, consistent with hip dysplasia and is noted to be similar to the opposite hip, as seen on postoperative radiographs. The patient was slowly returned to normal activity. Follow-up assessment was recommended at 6 months.

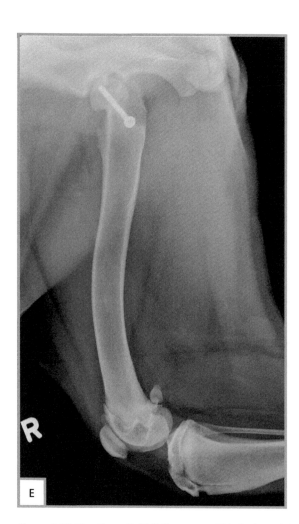

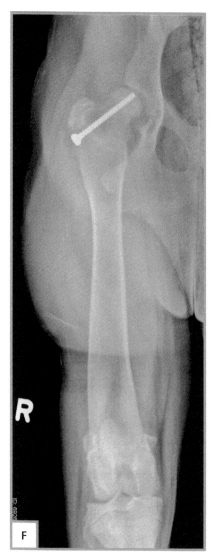

Figure 2.17 (Continued) (E) Follow-up at 4 Weeks: lateral view; (F) Follow-up at 4 Weeks: dorsal/ventral view.

Open, Grade II, Comminuted Fracture of the Femur

Signalment and History

A 5-year, 9-month-old, intact, female Laborador Retriever weighing 34 kg. She was found in a field with a gunshot wound near her right thigh 24 hours prior to presentation at the referral hospital. The wound was clipped and cleansed with systemic antibiotics administered within 8 hours of initial presentation.

Patient Assessment

The patient was in good physical condition.

Fracture Assessment

Open, grade II, comminuted fracture of the proximal fourth of the femur, displaced laterally (Figures 2.18A–B). The fracture appears consistent with that caused by a 22 caliber (0.22 of an inch) bullet. This size of bullet, given its muzzle velocity, can cause tissue damage, but not as severe as that caused by higher velocity rounds. Some references would classify this as an open, grade III fracture because it is a gunshot wound; however, there was minimal soft-tissue trauma. Worthy of note is that systemic antibiotics were initiated within hours of the trauma.

Options for Repair Methods

A locking plate plus rod fixation is the best choice for this fracture. Plating alone is unlikely to provide the required stiffness. This fracture allows for a questionable amount of proximal bone stock for the application of a DCP, and since an applied plate will act primarily as a buttress, a locking plate would be a good choice. An Interlocking nail could be considered, but the proximal section of bone is quite short for two transverse screws. IM pinning alone or external fixation would be inappropriate.

This was a gunshot wound with a high degree of comminution suggesting at least moderate energy imparted to the bone and soft tissue as well as a high likelihood of bone loss. Bone grafting should therefore be performed. At present, autogenous cancellous bone is considered the best choice for grafting. Bullet fragments should routinely be removed only if visible, in joints, impinging on the spinal cord or impinging on large nerves or nerve roots. Searching for and removing all bullet fragments is not necessary.

Surgery Report

An autogenous cancellous bone graft was obtained from the right proximal humerus. An approach to the shaft of the femur was performed. Care was taken to minimally disturb fracture fragments and soft tissues. The fracture was aligned using Kern bone-holding forceps to grasp the proximal and distal segments. The femur was not brought to the full length of the contralateral femur, but rather, under-reduced (but not more than by 20 percent) to minimize fracture gaps. A 4.76 mm Steinmann pin was normograded from the femoral intertrochanteric notch to the distal metaphysis. A 12-hole SOP locking plate was contoured to the lateral aspect of the femur and positioned, taking care to direct screws into both the proximal and distal metaphyses avoiding the IM pin. Sequentially, a screw was placed in screw hole 2, followed by screw hole 12. Screws were then placed in screw holes 1–3–9–10–11. The autogenous cancellous bone graft was placed in the area of comminution, concentrating on the medial aspect of the femur and gaps between bone fragments. A routine closure was performed.

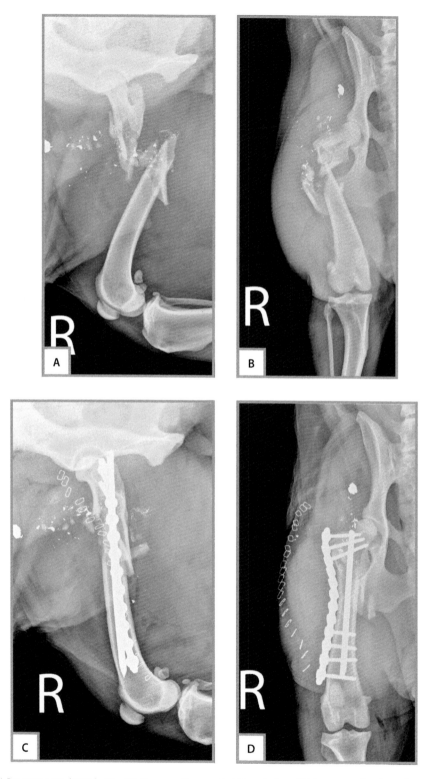

Figure 2.18 (A) Preoperative: lateral view; (B) Preoperative: ventral/dorsal view; (C) Postoperative: lateral view; (D) Postoperative: ventral/dorsal view.

(Continued)

Open, Grade II, Comminuted Fracture of the Femur *continued*

Postoperative Evaluation of Fracture Repair (Figures 2.18C–D)

Criteria	Assessment	Details
Alignment	Good	Overall bone alignment is achieved despite the comminution.
Apposition	Sufficient	The femur is not reduced to its original length. However, the femur can be shorted by 20 percent of its original length without causing lameness. Shortening was performed to reduce fracture gaps and subsequent non-union.
Apparatus	Sufficient	The IM pin should have been placed farther into the distal metaphysis. However, advancement is somewhat limited by the natural cranial bowing of the femur. Aggressive advancement may lead to penetration of the joint and damage to the patella. The SOP plate has only three screws in the proximal bone segment, which is all it would accommodate. Although the distal bone segment has four screws, a longer plate would have accommodated an additional one or two screws. A second plate would have been an option.

Follow-up at 8 Weeks (Figures 2.18E–F)

Criteria	Assessment
Alignment	Unchanged
Apposition	Unchanged
Apparatus	Unchanged
Activity	There is minimal callus formation at the fracture site. Although complete bone bridging circumferentially around the fracture site could not be identified radiographically, there appears to be isolated areas of bridging. Since healing is apparent, ancillary procedures such as an additional bone graft or the injection of PRP were not encouraged. Additional radiographs were recommended in 6 weeks. The patient was ambulating well and was thereafter lost to follow-up.

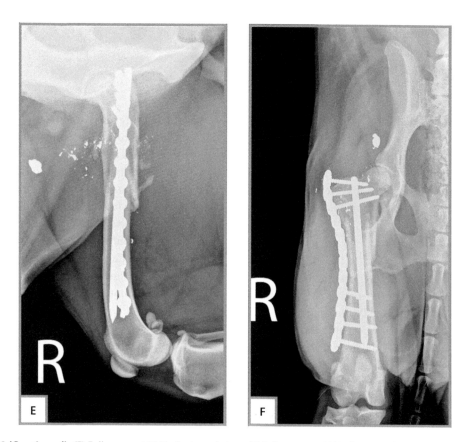

Figure 2.18 (Continued) (E) Follow-up at 8 Weeks: lateral view; (F) Follow-up at 8 Weeks: ventral/dorsal view.

Closed, Salter II Fracture of the Distal Femoral Physis

Signalment and History

A 5-month-old, recently neutered, female Bulldog weighing 13.6 kg was presented with fractures sustained from unknown trauma. The trauma was presumed to be from a motor vehicle accident based upon the patient having been found by the side of a road.

Patient Assessment

The patient was in sinus tachycardia on presentation, but heart rate returned to normal after the administration of IV fluids and pain medications. The patient was not in shock, but had sustained multiple injuries and abrasions consistent with being run over by a vehicle. Neurologic examination was within normal limits. There was potential for extensive soft tissue damage and devitalization of skin that may not be immediately apparent. There would be an increased risk of infection and potential for delayed healing. The patient's young age would be a positive prognostic indicator, as juvenile patients have faster and more robust healing.

Fracture Assessment

Closed, Salter II fracture of the left distal femoral physis, displaced caudally and medially with overriding of 1 cm. Closed, avulsion fracture of the left greater trochanter, displaced cranially 0.5 cm. Closed, incomplete transverse fracture of the left ilial shaft just caudal to the sacrum but with no displacement (Figures 2.19A–B).

Options for Repair Methods

The ilial shaft fracture should be treated conservatively. Even though it is technically in the weight-bearing segment of the pelvis, since it is not complete or displaced, it is stable and will quickly heal in this immature dog. The avulsion fracture of the greater trochanter is best treated with a tension band. This device will act to counter traction-forces, converting them to compressive forces along the fracture line. Although this will impede further growth from the proximal physis, aversive effects on clinical function are unlikely. Salter fractures of the distal femur are commonly Salter II with a metaphyseal fragment. This fragment, known as a Thurston-Holland fragment, can be large and complicate reduction/stabilization. Repair is commonly pins placed as cross pins or in Rush fashion. In dogs it is difficult to place pins in Rush fashion as the distal femur has a large cranial bow which may not allow the pins to advance to the proximal diaphysis within the medullary cavity. In most cases cross pins are employed. Alternative techniques reported include a single IM pin introduced from the intercondylar area or normograde placement of pins from the proximal femur.

Surgery Report

The patient was placed in the right lateral recumbent position. An approach to the distal femur and stifle joint through a lateral incision was performed. Care was taken not to elevate periosteum on the dorsal aspect of the metaphysis as these tissues can be used to assess fracture reduction. The distal femur was grasped with a Kern bone-holding forcep and the distal epiphysis grasped with pointed (Weber) bone-holding forceps. With traction and extension of the stifle, the fracture was reduced. The cartilage of the proximal trochlear groove was noted to be continuous with the periosteum of the metaphysis of the distal femur; suggesting proper reduction. A small 1.6 mm (14 gauge) Kirschner wire was placed from the origin of the caudal cruciate ligament across the physis for temporary stabilization of the fracture. A 2.0 mm IM pin was first introduced normograde from the origin of the long digital extensor tendon, angling less than 30 degrees to the long axis of the femur. It is reported that this angle or less can preserve growth of the femur from its distal

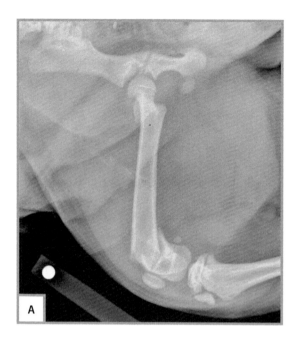

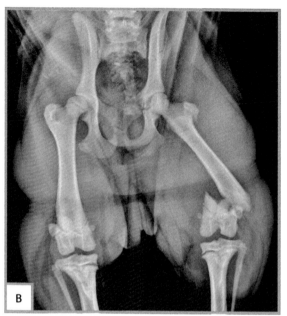

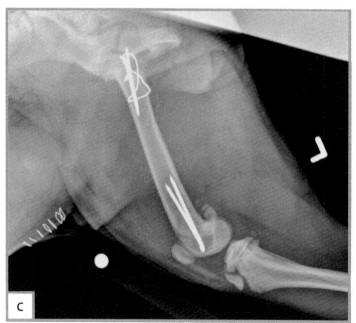

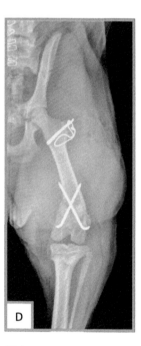

Figure 2.19 (A) Preoperative: lateral view; (B) Preoperative: ventral/dorsal view; (C) Postoperative: lateral view; (D) Postoperative: ventral/dorsal view.

(Continued)

Closed, Salter II Fracture of the Distal Femoral Physis *continued*

physis. A power drill was used with slow speed to prevent wobble and lessen heat production. The pin was advanced across the physis and into the metaphysis of the distal femur, stopping if the fracture began to displace medially. A second pin of the same diameter was introduced from the medial ephiphysis at a position similar to the previously used lateral landmark. The pins were advanced until they were minimally penetrating the transcortices of the distal femoral diaphysis. The pins were bent slightly, cut as close to the bone as possible, then further 'sunk' into the soft bone with a mallet and counter sink. The joint capsule and lateral fascia were closed in separate layers.

An approach to the craniodorsal aspect of the hip joint through a craniolateral incision was made but the coxofemoral joint was not entered. The avulsion fracture was identified and reduced. Two 1.6 mm Kirschner wires were placed from the greater trochanter into the proximal metaphysis of the femur perpendicular to the epiphysis and seated into the transcortex. A hole was drilled caudal-to-cranial across the proximal metaphysis using a Steinmann pin and 1 mm (18 gauge) cerclage wire was placed through the hole in a figure-of-eight pattern around the Kirschner wires. The wire was twisted tight. The Kirschner wires were bent dorsally and cut.

Postoperative Evaluation of Fracture Repair (Figures 2.19C–D)

Distal Femur

Criteria	Assessment	Details
Alignment	Good	The fracture is reduced adequately, though slightly under reduced by about 1 mm.
Apposition	Optimal	The fracture is reduced without a fracture gap.
Apparatus	Optimal	The pins are of an appropriate size and placed less than 30 degrees to the long axis of the femur. These pins cross well above the physis thus increasing the torsional stiffness of the repair without compromising epiphyseal bone growth. The pins minimally penetrate the far (trans) cortex. The pins are cut close to the metaphyseal bone and do not appear to impinge on soft tissues.

Greater Trochanter

Criteria	Assessment	Details
Alignment	Optimal	The greater trochanter is anatomically reduced.
Apposition	Optimal	The greater trochanter is compressed to the proximal femur by the resultant vector forces of the gluteal muscles and tension band.
Apparatus	Good	The tension band device appear adequately placed. The Kirschner wires are perpendicular to the physis, Sufficiently parallel to each other, and just minimally penetrate the far cortex. The cerclage wire is of adequate size and is anchored well in the metaphysis. The figure-of-eight wire crosses below the fracture line. There is only one twist on the cerclage wire. Though this may allow adequate tightening, the classic description is to use a twist on either side which will allow better tightening with greater compression.

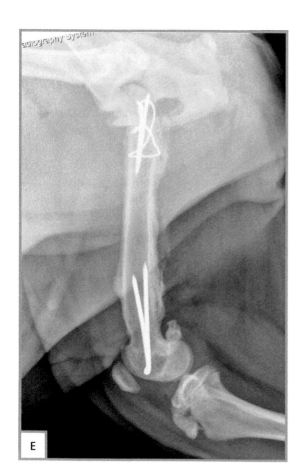

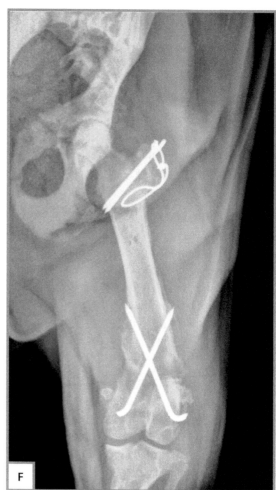

Figure 2.19 (Continued) (E) Follow-up at 7.5 Weeks: lateral view; (F) Follow-up at 7.5 Weeks: ventral/dorsal view.

Follow-up at 7.5 Weeks (Figures 2.19E–F)

Criteria	Assessment
Alignment	Unchanged
Apposition	Unchanged
Apparatus	Unchanged
Activity	
Distal femur	Good. The fracture appears healed. There is minimal callus at the fracture site, yet some callus is observed in the more proximal metaphyseal area.
Greater Trochanter	Optimal. The fracture appears healed.

Closed, Short Oblique Fracture of the Mid-Diaphysis of the Femur

Signalment and History

A 1-year, 5-month old, castrated, male Doberman Pinscher weighing 30 kg was presented to an emergency hospital following a motor vehicle accident. The vehicle was traveling at a moderate speed.

Patient Assessment

The patient was presented in shock and radiographs demonstrated a pneumothorax. Following resuscitation with intravenous fluids, electrocardiogram revealed ventricular premature contractions, but the patient was asymptomatic with normal blood pressure. The arrhythmia resolved after 24 hours.

Fracture Assessment

Closed, short, oblique fracture of the mid-diaphysis of the femur, displaced caudally and over-riding 3 cm (Figures 2.20A–B). This is a simple fracture in a good biological environment. Fracture healing should be uncomplicated as long as the fracture is adequately stabilized.

Options for Repair Methods

With this simple short oblique fracture, dynamic compression plating would be a very good option. If reduced with interfragmentary compression, load sharing or even dynamic compression should be achieved.

Cerclage wire cannot be used for this short, oblique fracture and IM pinning would not sufficiently oppose torsional forces. External fixation would not be optimal, even with a tie-in configuration, due to the size of the patient and the distance from connecting rod to bone which is long. Morbidity from pin tracts may also be a problem. Plate-rod configuration should be effective. However, if a locking plate were used in this simple fracture, high interfragmentary strain may negatively affect bone healing.

Surgery Report

A lateral approach to the shaft of the femur was made. The fracture was reduced with Kern bone-holding forceps. A 12-hole, 3.5 mm Broad LC-DCP plate was contoured to the lateral aspect of the femur. Screws were first placed into the distal bone fragment in screw holes 9 and 8, followed by screw hole 10. All screws were placed in neutral fashion. In screw holes 6 and 7, screws were placed at an angle through the plate and across the fracture line in lag fashion so as to impose compression across the oblique fracture line. The remaining screws were then placed. Closure was routine.

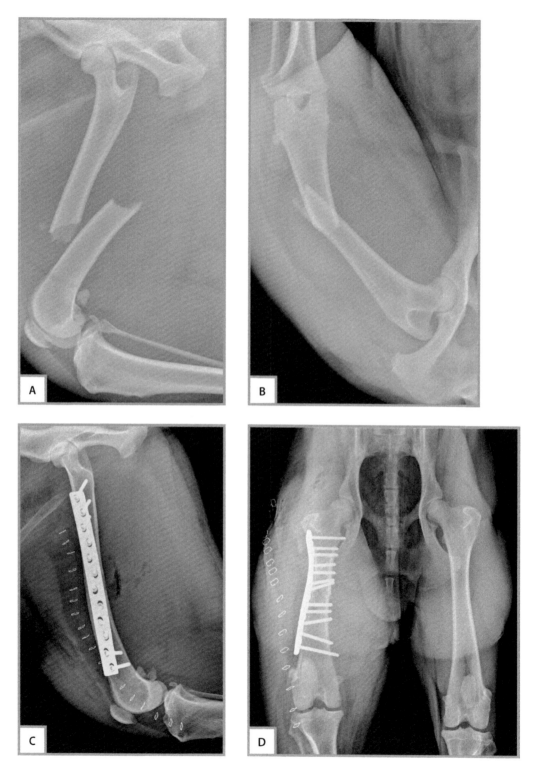

Figure 2.20 (A) Preoperative: lateral view; (B) Preoperative: cranial/caudal view; (C) Postoperative: lateral view; (D) Postoperative: cranial/caudal view.

(Continued)

Closed, Short Oblique Fracture of the Mid-Diaphysis of the Femur *continued*

Postoperative Evaluation of Fracture Repair (Figures 2.20C–D)

Criteria	Assessment	Details
Alignment	Optimal	The femur is reduced so that alignment of the joints and limb is anatomic.
Apposition	Sufficient	There is incomplete cortical contact on the medial aspect of the femur (transcortex, relative to the plate). As such, there may not be a medial buttress; however, a plate of this size should provide sufficient strength and stiffness for osteosynthesis. This repair may also allow some motion and a small fracture gap leading to high interfragmentary strain. The two screws crossing the fracture should limit this strain.
Apparatus	Optimal	The plate has been applied with proper technique, is sufficiently large and long enough for this size femur. There are more than sufficient screws on each side of the fracture (minimum of six engaged cortices).

Follow-up at 8 Weeks (Figures 2.20E–F)

Criteria	Assessment
Alignment	Unchanged
Apposition	Unchanged
Apparatus	Unchanged
Activity	There is modest-to-marked callus formation medially, cranially and caudally at the fracture site. Callus is bridging medially and cranially, but there is incomplete bridging caudally. The amount of callus and the presence of incomplete callus suggest motion and high interfragmentary strain. Although the plate is very stiff and the fracture gap is very small, slight motion can result in strains that may be too large for primary bone union. In addition, there were gaps on the medial cortex that may have been too large for primary bone union. The fracture had bridged on several aspects of the femur, the patient was ambulating well and the construct was intact. Even though it would have been desirous to perform additional radiographs in 4–6 weeks, the client was lost to follow-up.

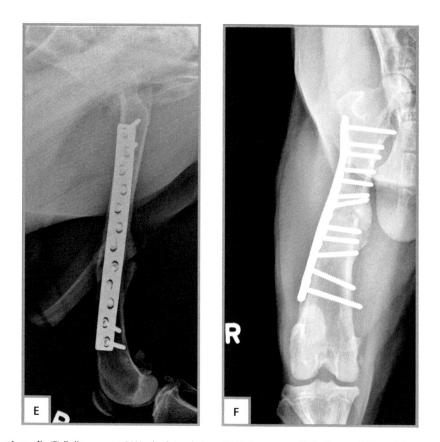

Figure 2.20 (Continued) (E) Follow-up at 8 Weeks: lateral view; (F) Follow-up at 8 Weeks: cranial/caudal view.

Closed, Salter II Fracture of the Distal Femur (Cat)

Signalment and History

A 9-month-old, castrated, male domestic, short-hair cat weighing 4 kg was presented with trauma of unknown origin to the right rear limb the day prior to presentation. The patient was slightly cachectic with a body score 4/10. There was a palpable fracture of the femur. Otherwise, no abnormalities were found on physical examination. The patient was an indoor cat and showed a calm demeanor.

Patient Assessment

This is a young cat with good capacity for bone healing. The patient's demeanor and home environment were favorable for bone healing.

Fracture Assessment

Closed, Salter II fracture of the distal femur, displaced laterally and not over-riding (Figures 2.21A–B). Fractures of the distal, femoral physis are most often Salter II fractures. These fractures should be operated soon after injury, as muscle contraction and fibrous tissue formation can make repair difficult if surgery is delayed longer than a few days.

Options for Repair Methods

Several pinning methods have been described including cross pinning, pins placed in Rush fashion, and a single IM pin from the distal epiphysis. Cats tend to have straight femurs; which makes the placement of pins in Rush fashion technically less challenging. The distal femoral physis has a W-shape and is relatively stable once reduced. It should be noted that an important aspect of fracture repair is the maintenance of a normal range of motion in the stifle. Young animals have an aggressive fibrous healing response. If the fracture is not repaired with attentive care to soft tissues, stabilized insufficiently or there is insufficient postoperative physical therapy, the healing callus can incorporate the quadriceps. This often leads to quadriceps contracture and a non-functional limb.

Surgery Report

An approach to the distal femur and stifle joint through a lateral incision was performed. The lateral superior genicular artery was ligated and the distal 3rd of the femur was exposed. The fracture was reduced being careful not to elevate periosteum at the proximal aspect of the trochlea groove as this periosteum can give indication of proper fracture reduction. The fracture was reduced by extending the stifle joint, after which the stifle joint was flexed while maintaining reduction. Pointed reduction forceps can be used to grasp the epiphysis, but care should be taken as the bone can be soft. A single 1.1 mm (17 gauge) Kirschner wire was placed across the physis and fracture starting at the origin of the caudal cruciate. This was a temporary wire. A 2.0 mm IM pin was drilled from the origin of the long digital extensor tendon at an approximate 20 degree angle to the long axis of the femur, crossing the physis and slightly into the metaphysis. A second pin of the same size was drilled from a comparable position on the medial aspect of the trochlear ridge. The pins were advanced until they were in the medullary cavity of the diaphysis. The pins were then withdrawn for removal of the trochar point that might penetrate cortical bone with further advancement. The pins were reinserted and advanced to the proximal femur. The pins were marked with a scalpel where they entered the distal femur, backed out and cut at the mark. They were then re-seated with a nail-set tool. The approach and arthrotomy were closed routinely, giving special attention to maintaining integrity of the lateral patellar-femoral ligament to prevent patellar luxation.

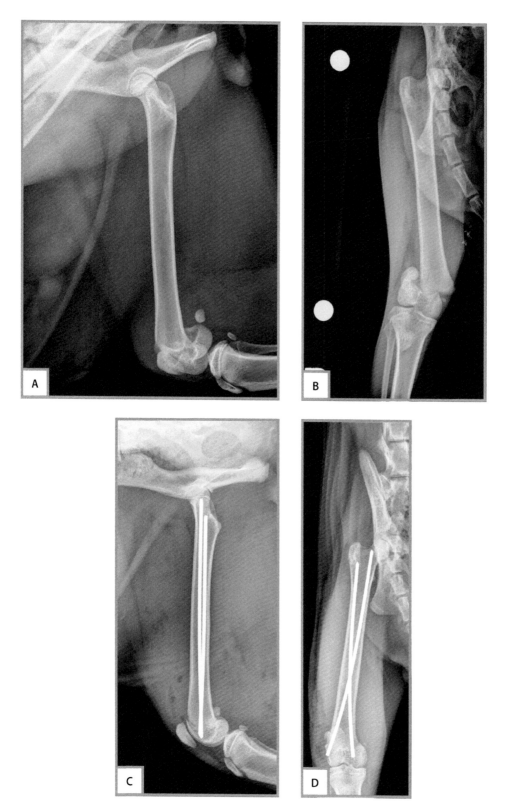

Figure 2.21 (A) Preoperative: lateral view; (B) Preoperative: cranial/caudal view; (C) Postoperative: lateral view; (D) Postoperative: cranial/caudal view.

(Continued)

Closed, Salter II Fracture of the Distal Femur *continued*

Postoperative Evaluation of Fracture Repair (Figures 2.21C–D)

Criteria	Assessment	Details
Alignment	Good	The alignment is sufficient, but slightly under-reduced. This is not uncommon with this type of fracture. Care should be taken to assure that the fracture is adequately reduced since it may appear reduced due to loss of periosteum at the proximal aspect of the trochlea.
Apposition	Optimal	The apposition is very good.
Apparatus	Optimal	The pins are of the correct size and were placed properly. The pins are at a sufficiently obtuse angle to the long axis of the femur and cross far above the physis. They are seated well into the metaphysis of the proximal femur.

Follow-up at 6 Weeks (Figures 2.21E–F)

Criteria	Assessment
Alignment	Unchanged
Apposition	Unchanged
Apparatus	Unchanged
Activity	The fracture has healed with minimal callus formation. The cat had excellent use of the limb and was returned to normal activity.

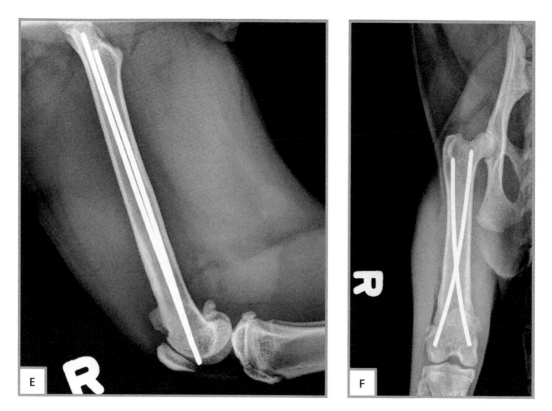

Figure 2.21 (Continued) (E) Follow-up at 6 Weeks: lateral view; (F) Follow-up at 6 Weeks: cranial/caudal view.

Closed, Salter II Fracture of the Distal Femur

Signalment and History
A 1-year-old, neutered, male Bichon Frise weighing 6 kg presented with a fractured right caudal limb following a jump from its owner's arms.

Patient Assessment
This is a young patient who sustained a relatively minor injury. There is good to excellent potential for healing.

Fracture Assessment
Closed Salter II fracture of the distal femur, displaced caudally, not over-riding. Fractures of the distal femoral physis are most often Salter II fractures. These fractures should be operated soon after injury, as muscle contraction and fibrous tissue formation can make repair difficult if surgery is delayed longer than a few days.

Options for Repair Methods
Several pinning methods have been described including cross pinning, pins placed in Rush fashion, and a single IM pin from the distal epiphysis. Dogs, especially of this breed, tend to have femurs which curve caudally, making rendering the placement of pins in Rush fashion technically difficult if not impossible. Cross pinning is commonly employed. The distal femoral physis has a W-shape and is relatively stable once reduced. It should be noted that an important aspect of fracture repair is maintenance of normal range of motion in the stifle. Young animals have an aggressive fibrous healing response. If the fracture is not repaired with attentive care to soft tissues; if the fracture is not stabilized sufficiently; or if there is insufficient postoperative physical therapy, the healing callus can incorporate the quadriceps. This often leads to quadriceps contracture and a non-functional limb.

Surgery Report
An approach to the distal femur and stifle joint through a lateral incision was performed. The lateral superior genicular artery was ligated and the distal 3rd of the femur was exposed. The fracture was reduced, being careful not to elevate periosteum at the proximal aspect of the trochlea groove as this periosteum can give indication of proper fracture reduction. The fracture was reduced by extending the stifle joint, after which the stifle joint was flexed while maintaining reduction. Pointed reduction forceps can be used to grasp the epiphysis, but care should be taken as the bone can be soft. A single 1.1 mm (17 gauge) Kirschner wire was placed across the physis and fracture starting at the origin of the caudal cruciate. This was a temporary wire. A 1.2 mm IM pin was drilled from the origin of the long digital extensor tendon at an approximate 30 degree angle to the long axis of the femur, crossing the physis and slightly into the metaphysis. A second pin of the same size was drilled from a comparable position on the medial aspect of the trochlear ridge. The pins were advanced until they exited the opposite cortexes. Drilling the pins alternatively prevents deviation of the epiphysis. The pins were marked with a scalpel where they entered the distal femur, backed out and cut at the mark. They were then re-seated with a nail set tool. The approach and arthrotomy were closed routinely, giving special attention to maintaining integrity of the lateral patellar-femoral ligament to prevent patellar luxation.

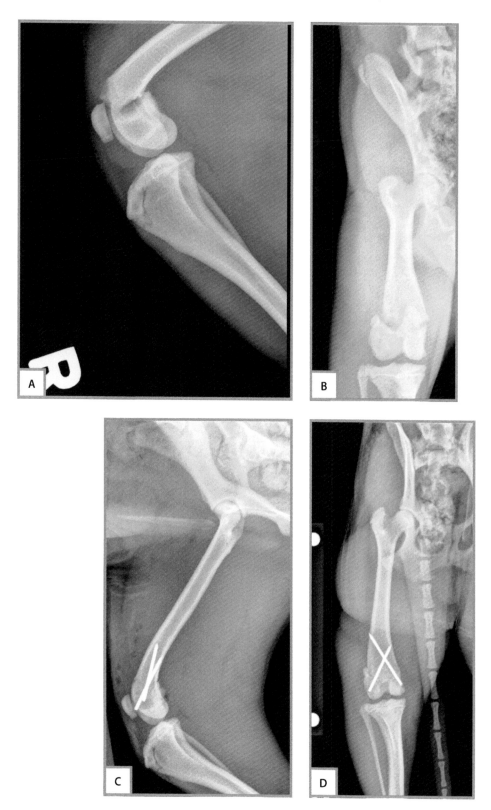

Figure 2.22 (A) Preoperative: lateral view; (B) Preoperative: cranial/caudal view; (C) Postoperative: lateral view; (D) Postoperative: cranial/caudal view.

(Continued)

Closed, Salter II Fracture of the Distal Femur *continued*

Post-operative Evaluation of Fracture Repair

Criteria	Assessment	Details
Alignment	Optimal	The fracture was anatomically reduced.
Apposition	Optimal	Fracture gaps are minimal.
Apparatus	Good	The pins cross well above the physis. It may have been possible to place the pins with less of an angle or place the pins in Rush fashion. The patient does not have any more growth from that physis, so these points may not be important.

Follow-up at 5 Weeks

Criteria	Assessment
Alignment	Unchanged
Apposition	Unchanged
Apparatus	Unchanged
Activity	The fracture has healed with minimal callus. The patient was returned to normal activity.

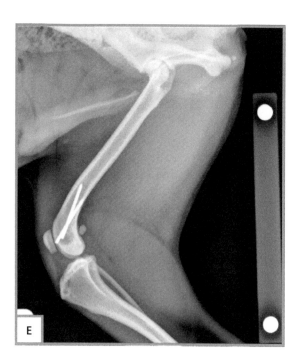

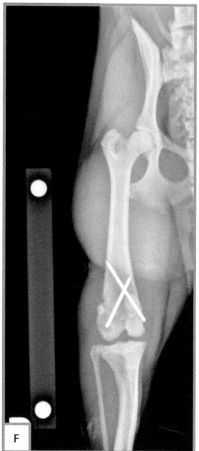

Figure 2.22 (Continued) (E) Follow-up at 5 Weeks: lateral view; (F) Follow-up at 5 Weeks: cranial/caudal view.

Closed, Tibial Tuberosity Avulsion

Signalment and History
A 5-month-old, Miniature Schnauzer weighing 6 kg sustained a fractured left rear limb after jumping from furniture. No other injuries were noted and the patient was in good health.

Patient Assessment
Very young patient with robust healing potential. There will be some continued growth of the caudal limbs.

Fracture Assessment
Closed, tibial tuberosity avulsion, displaced proximally 1 cm (Figures 2.23A–B). Tibial tuberosity fractures occur with some frequency, usually from falls. These carry a good prognosis; however, there will be compromise to growth of the tibial tuberosity.

Options for Repair Methods
Tibial tuberosity fractures are commonly repaired with tension band fixation. Pull of the quadriceps is countered by the tension band, resulting in compression of the tibial tuberosity to the proximal tibia. This is a highly successful surgery for subsequent healing; however, continued growth of the tibial tuberosity is arrested. Physis of the tibial plateau continues to grow. As it grows the straight patellar tendon may not lengthen and the patella is pulled in a more distal or low position known as patella baja. In most cases this is not a concern except when the injury occurs in an immature dog of a large breed. Under these conditions, the tibial tuberosity may need to be repositioned to a more normal position as the patient reaches skeletal maturity.

Surgery Report
The patient was placed in the dorsal recumbent position and a medial approach to the proximal tibia was performed. The tibia was digitally reduced and a 1.2 mm (16 gauge) Kirschner wire was placed through the tibial tuberosity into the metaphysis of the proximal tibia to the length of the caudal cortex. A second wire was placed in a similar manner lateral to the first wire. A hole was made transversely in the cranial tibia 1.5 times the distance from the pins to the cranial fracture so the final figure-of-eight wire would cross distal to the fracture line. A loop was made in a section of 0.8 mm (20 gauge) cerclage wire. The short end of the wire was passed through the hole from medial-to-lateral while the long end was brought laterally to encircle the Kirschner wires before again being brought lateral. The two wire ends were then twisted together. Both this twist and the original wire loop were alternately pulled while twisting until the tension band wire was taught. The cerclage wire twists were cut, leaving no less than two complete twists, after which the remaining wire 'stumps' were bent to reside closely adjacent to the tibial cortex. The Kirschner wires were bent proximally as much as possible and cut. The incision was closed routinely.

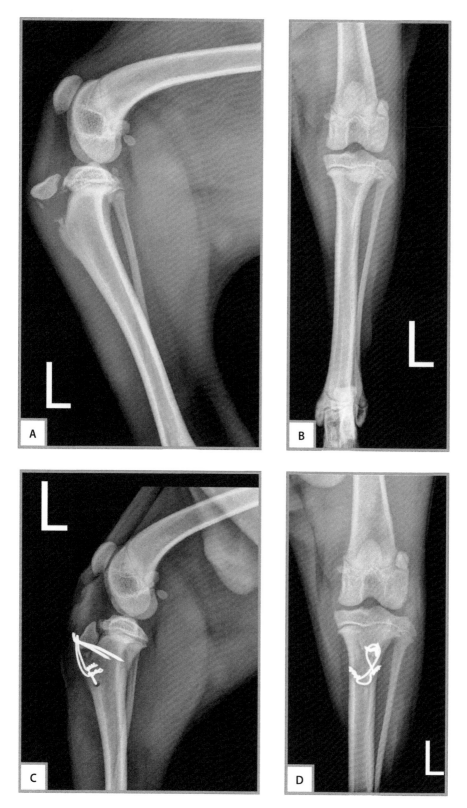

Figure 2.23 (A) Preoperative: lateral view; (B) Preoperative: cranial/caudal view; (C) Postoperative: lateral view; (D) Postoperative: cranial/caudal view.

(Continued)

Closed, Tibial Tuberosity Avulsion *continued*

Postoperative Evaluation of Fracture Repair (Figures 2.23C–D)

Criteria	Assessment	Details
Alignment	Optimal	The tibial tuberosity is anatomically repositioned.
Apposition	Sufficient	The fracture line will not be completely reduced as this is a physis.
Apparatus	Sufficient	The Kirschner wires and cerclage wire are of appropriate size. The Kirschner wires engage the tibial tuberosity, but could have been inserted more proximal to engage more of the tuberosity while not impinging on the straight patellar tendon. The cerclage wire crosses correctly relative to the fracture line and the twists are around one another, rather than one wire twisted around the other; allowing the cerclage to slip. The twists are placed next to the bone.

Follow-up at 5 Weeks (Figures 2.23E–F)

Criteria	Assessment
Alignment	Unchanged
Apposition	The epiphyseal physis has closed.
Apparatus	There may be some backing out of the Kirschner wires, which is not uncommon.
Activity	The epiphyseal physis has closed, and there is continued growth of the tibial tuberosity resulting in a mild, distal residence of the patella. In this patient there is no need to reposition the tibial tuberosity without abnormal clinical function. Continued migration of implants or soft tissue irritation from the implants may require implant removal.

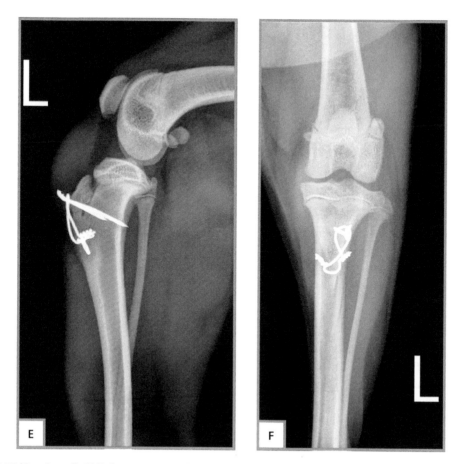

Figure 2.23 (Continued) (E) Follow-up at 5 Weeks: lateral view; (F) Follow-up at 5 Weeks: cranial/caudal view.

Closed, Spiral, Long Oblique Fracture of the Left Tibia

Signalment and History
A 2-year-old, neutered, female Labrador Retriever weighing 37 kg sustained a left rear limb injury from a motor vehicle accident. In addition, there were numerous abrasions on the carpi, head, and left lateral stifle. Thoracic and abdominal radiographs were within normal limits. Capillary refill time was greater than 3 seconds. Intravenous fluids and analgesics were administered, and a Robert Jones bandage was applied to the left rear limb. The patient was referred to the surgical service the following day.

Patient Assessment
The patient presented in a mild state of shock, but responded well to fluid therapy. The abrasions on the forelimbs as well as injury to the caudal limb suggested a noteworthy degree of trauma. Though the thoracic radiographs were within normal limits on presentation, the patient was monitored closely for trauma coincident to that involving the pelvic limb. Otherwise this was a healthy patient that responded well to initial therapy and had a good prognosis for recovery to the rear limb injury.

Fracture Assessment
Closed, spiral, long oblique fracture to the mid-shaft of the left tibia, displaced laterally, over-riding 5 mm with a large butterfly fragment. The fibula is fractured but not displaced. The spiral oblique fracture does not suggest high-energy impact trauma (Figures 2.24A–B).

Options for Repair Methods
External splinting or casting could be considered. However, as the fracture is long oblique and with some comminution, shear forces across the fracture site would be high and surgical internal fixation would be preferred. A long oblique fracture can be repaired by several methods. An IM pin or nail with cerclage wire of the long oblique fracture would be a simple and appropriate choice. External fixation using a bilateral, Type II fixator, with or without cerclage wires of the fracture would also be an appropriate choice, as would MIPO.

Surgery Report
Three separate 3 cm incisions were made. Firstly at the medial aspect of the proximal, second center, and third at the distal tibia. The proximal tibia was reamed in preparation for normograde placement of an IM nail. An interlocking nail, 185 mm long, 6 mm diameter was placed normograde within the medullary cavity and was visually observed to continue into the distal tibia from the center incision. The third, then fourth bolts were placed using an aiming device. Reduction and rotational alignment was visually confirmed. The first and second bolts were then placed. Fracture gaps and fissures were observed at the fracture site. An autogenous cancellous bone graft was obtained from the greater tubercle of the left humerus and placed in the fracture area. The incisions were closed routinely.

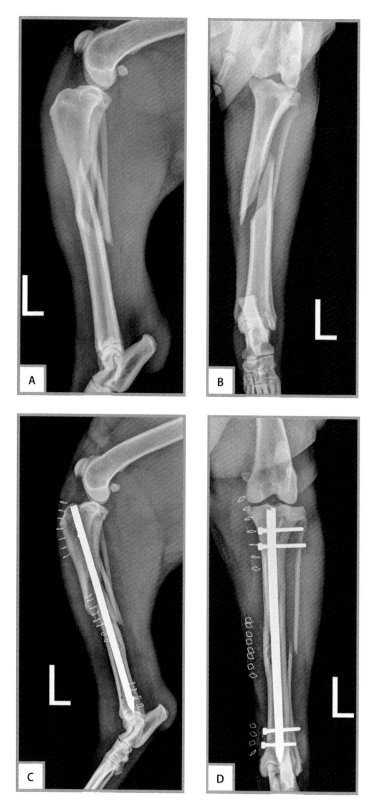

Figure 2.24 (A) Preoperative: lateral view; (B) Preoperative: cranial/caudal view; (C) Postoperative: lateral view; (D) Postoperative: cranial/caudal view.

(Continued)

Closed, Spiral, Long Oblique Fracture of the Left Tibia *continued*

Postoperative Evaluation of Fracture Repair (Figures 2.24C–D)

Criteria	Assessment	Details
Alignment	Optimal	The tibia is reduced to normal anatomic alignment.
Apposition	Sufficient	Fracture lines contained gaps, and additional fractures and fissures (not appreciated on preoperative radiographs) became radiographically apparent.
Apparatus	Sufficient	The IM nail appears to occupy the entire medullary canal and may obstruct medullary blood supply. The distal nail is too close to the articular cartilage of the tibial tarsal joint. The length of the two proximal bolts are too long.

Follow-up at 8 Weeks (Figures 2.24E–F)

Criteria	Assessment
Alignment	Unchanged
Apposition	Unchanged
Apparatus	Unchanged
Activity	Moderate callus is present throughout the fractured area. Though fracture lines can be visualized, the callus bridged all sides of the tibia. The patient was slowly returned to normal activity.

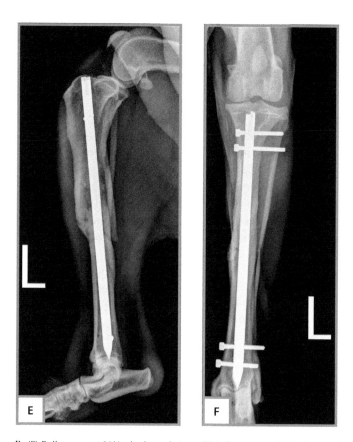

Figure 2.24 (Continued) (E) Follow-up at 8 Weeks: lateral view; (F) Follow-up at 8 Weeks: cranial/caudal view.

Closed, Comminuted Fracture of the Mid-to-Distal 3rd of the Tibia

Signalment and History
A 2-year-old, intact, male Labrador Retriever weighing 35 kg was admitted with a fractured tibia sustained by falling from a height of several feet. The patient was initially taken to a veterinary hospital where a Robert Jones bandage and analgesics were administered and was thereafter presented for fracture fixation the following day.

Patient Assessment
This is a low-energy injury in a relatively young patient. Inherently, the tibia (particularly distal) does not have a robust blood supply due to scant muscle cover and therefore is associated with a relatively high incidence of delayed- or non-unions. However, in this patient the healing potential appears good since the periosteum is likely intact.

Fracture Assessment
Closed, comminuted fracture with short oblique fracture lines of the mid-to-distal 3rd of the tibia, minimally displaced and not over-riding (Figures 2.25A–B). The fracture is minimally displaced, and the fibula is intact. The nature of this fracture was low-energy. All these factors contribute to a good-to-excellent environment for healing.

Options for Repair Methods
This fracture could be treated with external support of a cast and splint. However, this approach mandates the need for meticulous bandage care, which may be difficult for this age and breed. An external fixator could be successfully used if applied closed and would be an acceptable choice in this conjecturally rapid-healing fracture. The patient and apparatus would require daily assessment. Open reduction and internal fixation with dynamic plate fixation would compromise the presumptive intact periosteum. It is possible that the comminuted segments could not be reduced with interfragmenary compression and load sharing would not be achieved, negating any benefit of the exposure. MIPO with a locking plate and IM pin could be performed to maintain an optimal biologic environment of the fracture area, as well as provide adequate mechanical support in strength and stiffness. Such fixation would not require the need for an external construct. Since the fibula is intact, it will serve as an auxiliary lateral fixation support.

Surgery Report
The patient was placed in the dorsal recumbent position. Two medial incisions were made. Firstly a 2 cm incision, 1 cm distal to the tibial plateau and distal to the medial collateral ligament. The second was also 2 cm in length, but 1 cm proximal to the medial maleolus. A periosteal elevator was used to create a supraperiosteal path connecting the two incisions; a path close to the medial bone cortex, but not invading the periosteum. A 12-hole, 3.5 mm locking, compression plate was contoured based on radiographs of the contralateral tibia. The plate was introduced into the proximal incision, tracking along the medial bone surface until visualized at the distal incision. Limb alignment was visually assessed. A locking screw was placed in screw hole 2. A second screw was placed in screw hole 11. Limb alignment was again visually assessed, then screws were placed in sequence in screw holes 1–3–10–12. The incisions were closed routinely.

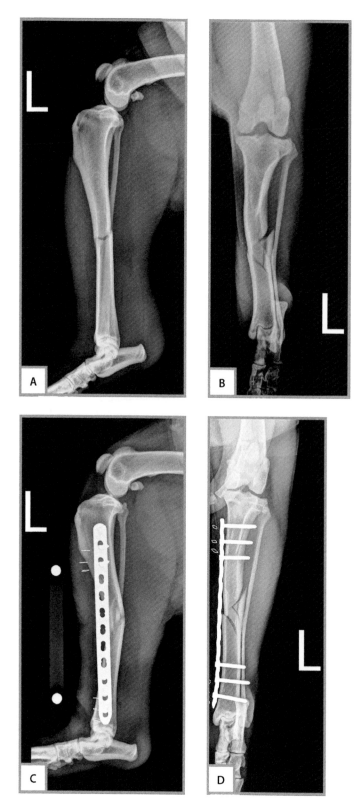

Figure 2.25 (A) Preoperative: lateral view; (B) Preoperative: cranial/caudal view; (C) Postoperative: lateral view; (D) Postoperative: cranial/caudal view.

(Continued)

Closed, Comminuted Fracture of the Mid-to-Distal 3rd of the Tibia *continued*

Postoperative Evaluation of Fracture Repair (Figures 2.25C–D)

Criteria	Assessment	Details
Alignment	Sufficient	There is mild angulation on the medial to lateral plane. There is also moderate caudal angulation. It is possible that there is internal rotation as suggested by the position of the calcaneous on the cranial-caudal radiograph. This was not appreciated visually or on the lateral radiograph. Reduction in the medial-to-lateral plane is most important in the tibia to ensure proper joint articulation. Since the hock and stifle are hinge joints (ginglymus), angulation in the medial-to-lateral plane from inaccurate reduction cannot be compensated by changes in joint angles. Accordingly, the distal limb will deviate medially or laterally, depending on the malalignment. In contrast, some malalignment in the cranial-to-caudal plane is tolerated by compensatory bending at the joint. Similar to a tibial plateau leveling operation, modest angulation is tolerated without abnormal limb carriage or lameness. Finally, rotational malalignment is not well tolerated, and if present (as in this case), is mild and goes clinically unnoticed.
Apposition	Good	The fracture had moderately large fracture gaps but the intent of this procedure was not to eliminate them. Noting that the biological environment at the fracture site was considered good, better apposition was not considered critical.
Apparatus	Good	The plate was placed reasonably close to the bone. There are three screws at both the proximal and distal ends of the plate and the plate spans a long length of the bone. Some screws are seen exiting the trans-cortex by several millimeters, but are unlikely to cause soft tissue irritation. This plate in this 35 kg patient would be insufficient sole fixation if the fibula were not intact. If the fibula were fractured, an IM pin should have been added to the fixation.

Follow-up at 5 Weeks (Figures 2.25E–F)

Criteria	Assessment
Alignment	Unchanged
Apposition	Unchanged
Apparatus	Unchanged
Activity	New bone is forming at the fracture lines and bridges the bone segments both laterally and caudally. Bone does not appear to have bridged the fracture site medially and could not be visualized cranially due to the location of the plate. The bone is healing as anticipated and the owner did not return for subsequent radiographic follow-up.

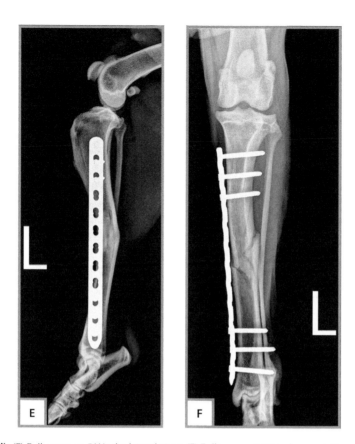

Figure 2.25 (Continued) (E) Follow-up at 5 Weeks: lateral view; (F) Follow-up at 5 Weeks: cranial/caudal view.

Closed, Malunion of a Left Mid-Tibia and Mid-Fibula Fracture

Signalment and History
A 4-month-old, intact, female Abyssinian-mix cat weighing 2 kg was presented for evaluation of a crooked limb.

Patient Assessment
The patient was recently adopted but in good health.

Fracture Assessment
Closed, malunion of a left mid-tibia and mid-fibula fracture, the distal segment is displaced laterally without deviation in the cranial caudal plane or over-riding (Figures 2.26A–B). This malunion occurred long before presentation and has healed. Malunions in the medial lateral plan are not well tolerated, as they place abnormal forces on the adjacent stifle and hock hinge joints. Correction of the deformity is warranted. This young cat has great healing potential.

Options for Repair Methods
The tibia and fibula will need to be osteotomized. Often, a closing wedge osteotomy is performed to correct the angular deformity, followed by stabilization with internal fixation. Plate fixation should be considered and dynamic compression plating of the osteotomy would allow reduction with compression. External fixation should also be considered, wherein, initially, two proximal and distal fixator pins can be used to reduce the osteotomy and align the limb.

Surgery Report
An approach to the shaft of the tibia was performed. A 2.0 mm positive-profile end-threaded pin was placed perpendicular to the proximal diaphysis 1.5 cm distal to the tibial plateau. A second 2.0 mm end-threaded pin was placed perpendicular to the distal diaphysis 1 cm proximal to the medial malleolus. At the area of greatest tibial angulation, an osteotomy was made perpendicular to the proximal diaphysis and parallel to the proximal fixator pin. The fibula was also osteotomized. A second osteotomy was performed in the distal segment close to the first and perpendicular to the distal tibia, paralleling the fixator pins. The fixator pins were positioned parallel to one another and connected to a 3.2 mm connecting rod. Reduction was visually inspected and two additional fixator pins were placed 1 cm from the osteotomy. The incision was closed routinely.

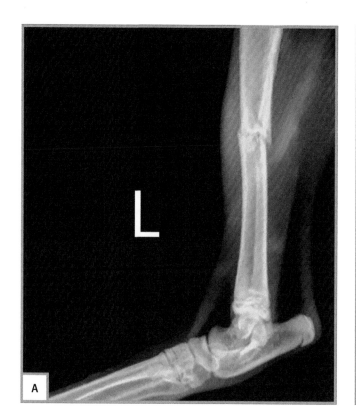

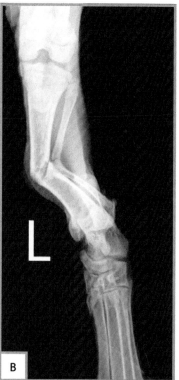

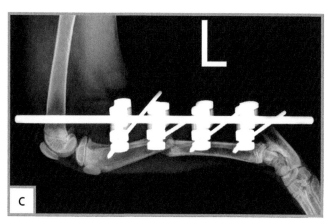

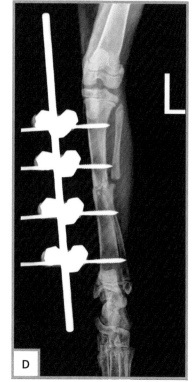

Figure 2.26 (A) Preoperative: lateral view; (B) Preoperative: cranial/caudal view; (C) Postoperative: lateral view; (D) Postoperative: cranial/caudal view.

(Continued)

Closed, Malunion of a Left Mid-Tibia and Mid-Fibula Fracture *continued*

Postoperative Evaluation of Fracture Repair (Figures 2.26C–D)

Criteria	Assessment	Details
Alignment	Sufficient	Angulation on the medial-to-lateral plane was corrected and no rotational malformation was created. There is some caudal bowing at the osteotomy in the cranial caudal plane.
Apposition	Sufficient	There is some cranial translation of the distal segment, but intrafracture contact of the diaphysis is greater than 50 percent; a criterion for adequate reduction.
Apparatus	Sufficient	Though this is a small patient, this fixator is also rather small. A larger connecting rod or bilateral construct could have been considered. Since there is cortical contact at the area of the osteotomy, there should be load sharing between the bone and construct; therefore, the fixator need not bear the entire axial load of weight bearing. An additional fixator pin could have been considered in each of the two bone segments, but that would have added to the overall weight of the fixator in this small patient.

Follow-up at 10 Weeks (Figures 2.26E–F)

Criteria	Assessment
Alignment	Unchanged
Apposition	Unchanged
Apparatus	Unchanged and all pins are secure.
Activity	Recheck examination was requested at 4 weeks. At this time there is mature bone healing and bridging on all aspects of the osteotomy. The callus is beginning to remodel and the tibia is beginning to remodel into a straighter configuration. The fixator was removed (see Figures 26G–H) and the cat returned to normal activity.

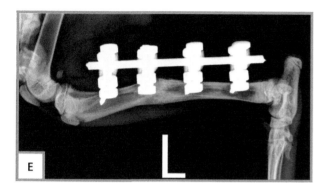

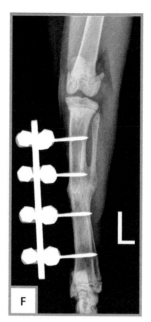

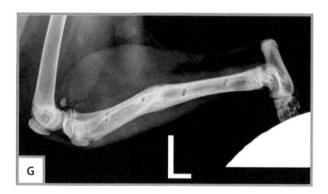

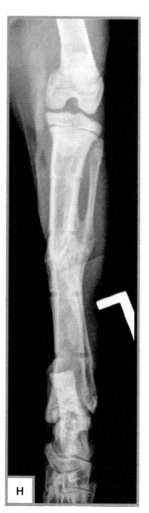

Figure 2.26 (Continued) (E) Follow-up at 10 Weeks: lateral view; (F) Follow-up at 10 Weeks: cranial/caudal view; (G) Following fixator removal: lateral view; (H) Following fixator removal: cranial/caudal view.

Closed, Highly Comminuted Fracture of the Tibia

Signalment and History

A 9-year-old, neutered, male Standard Poodle weighing 33 kg sustained a tibial fracture from a motor vehicle accident.

Patient Assessment

The patient presented in shock and was administered intravenous fluids. Thoracic radiograph demonstrated pulmonary contusions and a mild pneumothorax. Abdominal radiographs and neurologic examination were within normal limits. The tibia was placed in a Robert Jones bandage and the patient was transferred the following day to the surgical center.

Fracture Assessment

Closed, highly comminuted fracture of the tibia, with comminution extending from the proximal 4th to the distal 4th of the diaphysis; displaced cranially, over-riding 1.5 cm. The fibula was fractured at the proximal 4th and mid-diaphysis (Figures 2.27A–B). This is a high-energy fracture as demonstrated by the degree of comminution and displacement. The tibia has minimal soft tissue cover at its mid-to-distal section, thereby providing a less than optimal biological environment for fracture healing, resulting in an area subject to delayed- or non-union. Efforts should be made to preserve and/or enhance this microenvironment in addition to providing a strong and stiff fixation construct.

Options for Repair Methods

External support would not be appropriate. The comminution has components that are short and oblique; therefore, fracture reconstruction with cerclage wire would not be appropriate. Further, it is unlikely that the fracture could be reconstructed with techniques such as lag screws. Non- or minimally-invasive techniques would be most appropriate. An interlocking nail should be considered, but the distal segment may not allow two screws or bolts. External fixation with a Type II or bilateral fixator should be considered. This could be applied without an approach to the fracture site. Such a fixator would need to be maintained, but could be adjusted in stiffness as the fracture heals. MIPO could be considered. Noteworthy, is a short, 3 cm, distal fracture segment that may not allow placement of three distal screws. A locking plate system should therefore be considered. A non-locking DCP placed in buttress fashion may be suitable but would require precise contouring and lack the offering of angle-stable screws. With plate fixation technique, an IM pin should be used to increase the strength and stiffness of the construct. Considering the age of the patient, a bone graft should also be considered for placement in the areas of fracture gaps.

Surgery Report

The patient was placed in the dorsal recumbent position and a 4 cm incision was made starting at the medial aspect of the tibial plateau. A second, 2 cm, incision was made 1 cm proximal to the medial maleolus. A 3.2 mm IM pin was normograded from the proximal tibial plateau and seated into the distal tibial metaphysis. After starting placement of this pin, it was removed, the tip was blunted and then reintroduced into the same guide hole and seated. After seating, the pin was marked at the level of the tibial plateau, withdrawn, cut at that mark, and again seated, this time with a counter sink. A 15-hole, 3.5 mm broad, LC-DCP was contoured compliant to radiographs of the contralateral tibia. A periosteal elevator was used to create plate passage subperiosteal from the proximal-to-distal incision. The first and fifteenth screws were placed bicortically, after which fracture reduction was confirmed. Bicortical screws were placed in sequence in screw holes 2, 3 and 14. Unicortical screws were placed in holes 4 and 5. Bone grafting was not performed. The incision was closed routinely. Postoperative radiographs revealed that the third bicortical screw entered the fracture line. This screw, as well as those in screw holes 4 and 5 were replaced with 4.0 mm cancellous screws. The screw in hole 1 was redirected. (postoperative radiographs not shown).

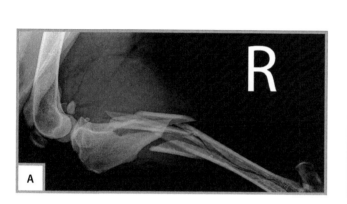

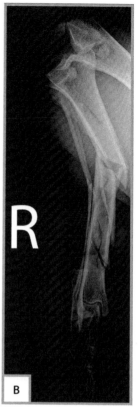

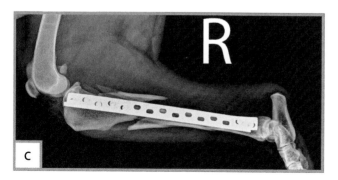

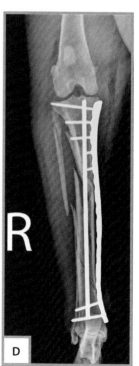

Figure 2.27 (A) Preoperative: lateral view; (B) Preoperative: cranial/caudal view; (C) Postoperative: lateral view; (D) Postoperative: cranial/caudal view.

(Continued)

Closed, Highly Comminuted Fracture of the Tibia *continued*

Postoperative Evaluation of Fracture Repair (Figures 2.27C–D)

Criteria	Assessment	Details
Alignment	Good	There is very good alignment in the cranial-to-caudal plane. There is slight medial bowing in the medial-to-lateral plane.
Apposition	Sufficient	There are relatively large interfragmentary gaps laterally at the proximal 4th of the fracture. Fracture gaps in the remainder of the diaphysis are small; suggesting an intact periosteum.
Apparatus	Sufficient	The pin is of appropriate size for a plate/rod construct. A locking plate may have been preferred; however, a locking, broad, 3.5 mm plate was not immediately available at the time of surgery. Screws are angle stable and perpendicular in many locking plate systems and these may have directed the proximal screw toward the joint; allowing only unicortical purchase in the small proximal segment. There was a need for unicortical screws as these have a far greater utility in locking plates compared to non-locking plates. Radiographs suggest the first (and possibly second) screws transit the head of the fibula. This is undesirable, as it may result in painful ambulation. Distally, the fracture line allowed placement of only two screws. It would be advised to radiograph this fracture at an early postoperative date to observe the course of healing, integrity of implants, and to determine if subsequent bone healing stimulation is warranted.

First Follow-up at 6 Weeks (Figures 2.27E–F)

Criteria	Assessment
Alignment	Unchanged
Apposition	Unchanged
Apparatus	Unchanged
Activity	There is periosteal activity suggesting active healing. There is also modest callus formation in the areas of the proximal fracture lines suggesting healing is slow, but is progressing. As the fixation was stable and progressively healing, no additional surgical procedures were recommended and a recheck in 4 weeks was scheduled.

Final Follow-up at 10 Weeks (Figures 2.27G–H)

Criteria	Assessment
Alignment	Unchanged
Apposition	Unchanged
Apparatus	Unchanged
Activity	Although fracture lines are still present, there is circumferential bridging callus, suggesting osteosynthesis. The patient was slowly returned to normal activity.

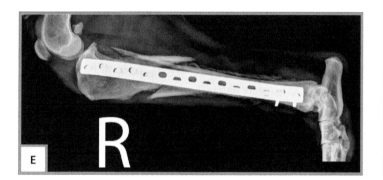

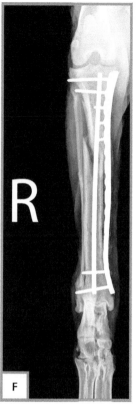

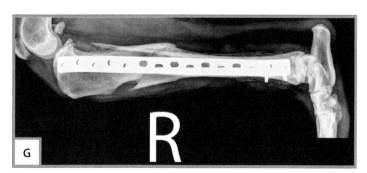

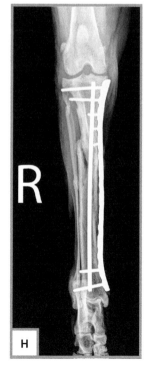

Figure 2.27 (Continued) (E) First Follow-up at 6 Weeks: lateral view; (F) First Follow-up at 6 Weeks: cranial/caudal view; (G) Final Follow-up at 10 Weeks: lateral view; (H) Final Follow-up at 10 Weeks: cranial/caudal view.

Closed, Long Oblique Fracture of the Right Tibia

Signalment and History
A 2-year, 8-month-old, intact, female Boxer weighing 22 kg sustained a tibia fracture falling downstairs. She was presented to the referral hospital the same day.

Patient Assessment
The patient was in good condition and the limb was placed in a Robert Jones bandage soon after the injury. She was considered a good candidate for surgery and bone healing.

Fracture Assessment
Closed, long, oblique fracture of the distal 3rd of the right tibia with one large fragment (Figures 2.28A–B).

Options for Repair Methods
The fracture is considered a long oblique fracture when including the length of the fragment. This allows the fracture to be cerclaged, however, ancillary fixation must also be used, such as a plate. This can be either a locking or DCP. Use of an IM pin as the ancillary device could be considered, but the fracture is sufficiently distal that a pin may not counter bending forces. An interlocking nail or external fixation with or without cerclage wires would be a good option, but would not be as stable as cerclage wire plus plate fixation. A plate placed in minimally invasive fashion could also be considered. The attributes of interlocking nail or external fixation, without cerclage wires, are attractive as they can be applied using minimally invasive techniques. External coaptation would not be a good option because the distal tibia has a poor blood supply and oblique fractures can develop high shear forces.

Surgery Report
An approach to the medial shaft of the tibia was performed, placing a Penrose drain around the saphenous artery and nerve for ease of retraction during surgery. The three fracture segments were reduced using Kern bone-holding forceps or pointed bone-holding forceps. Four, 1 mm (18 gauge) cerclage wires were placed 12 mm apart (the distance between screw holes in a standard 3.5 mm DCP). An 11-hole 3.5 mm LC-DCP plate was contoured to the medial tibia and placed so that the cerclage wires were between screw holes. Screws placed in screw holes 3 and 10 were placed in neutral fashion. The remaining screws were then applied. Screw holes 7 and 8 were left open because fracture lines were underlying these holes. The approach was closed routinely.

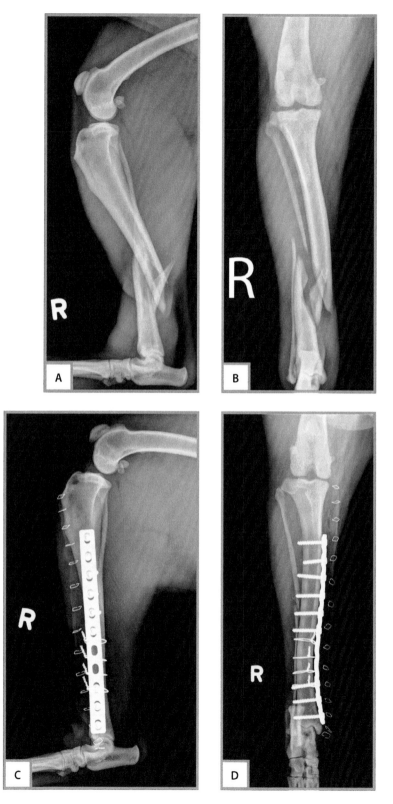

Figure 2.28 (A) Preoperative: lateral view; (B) Preoperative: cranial/caudal view; (C) Postoperative: lateral view; (D) Postoperative: cranial/caudal view.

(Continued)

Closed, Long Oblique Fracture of the Right Tibia *continued*

Postoperative Evaluation of Fracture Repair (Figures 2.28C–D)

Criteria	Assessment	Details
Alignment	Optimal	The fracture is anatomically reduced; restoring the original conformation of the tibia.
Apposition	Optimal	The fracture fragments are compressed using the cerclage wires.
Apparatus	Good	The correct number and position of cerclage wires were used. Some surgeons prefer loop cerclage wires, as some studies suggest they can be placed more tightly than twisted cerclage wires. The fourth cerclage wire closure may be of concern, as it is close to screw 9. The cerlage wires should have been cut shorter with 2-4 complete twists. The plate is placed appropriately with six cortices engaged in the distal bone segment.

First Follow-up at 6 Weeks (Figures 2.28E–F)

Criteria	Assessment
Alignment	Unchanged
Apposition	Unchanged
Apparatus	Unchanged
Activity	There is minimal callus formation, suggesting the fracture is healing with primary bone union; however, fracture lines can still be seen radiographically.

Final Follow-up at 11 Weeks (Figures 2.28G–H)

Criteria	Assessment
Alignment	Unchanged
Apposition	Unchanged
Apparatus	Unchanged
Activity	There is still minimal-to-no callus formation, suggesting the fracture is, indeed, healing with primary bone union. Fracture lines are no longer apparent.

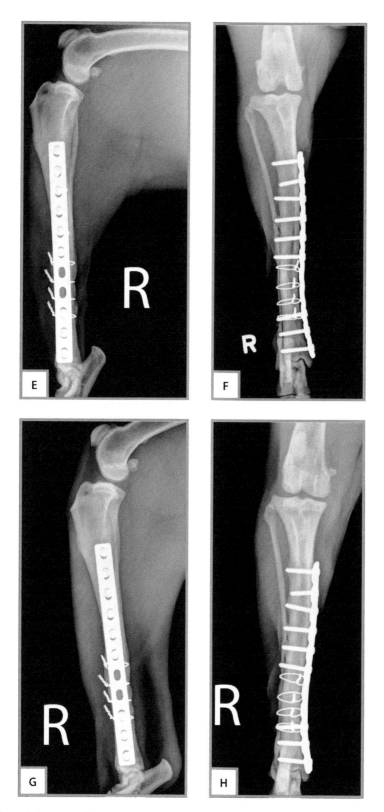

Figure 2.28 (Continued) (E) First Follow-up at 6 Weeks: lateral view; (F) First Follow-up at 6 Weeks: cranial/caudal view; (G) Final Follow-up at 11 Weeks: lateral view; (H) Final Follow-up at 11 Weeks: cranial/caudal view.

Closed, Highly Comminuted Fracture of the Mid-to-Distal 4th of the Tibia

Signalment and History
A 2-year-old, neutered, female Siberian Husky weighing 21 kg sustained a right tibial fracture from a motor vehicle accident. The patient was presented to an emergency clinic in good condition where she was administered intravenous fluids and the limb was placed in a Robert Jones bandage.

Patient Assessment
Thoracic and abdominal radiographs were within normal limits. The patient is relatively young with good healing potential and was otherwise in good condition without significant soft tissue trauma.

Fracture Assessment
Closed, highly comminuted fracture of the mid-to-distal 4th of the tibia, mildly displaced laterally and over-riding 5 mm. The fibula is also fractured in the adjacent area. Although comminuted, the fracture is minimally displaced and with the periosteum likely intact (Figures 2.29A–B).

Options for Repair Methods
External support with a cast or splint could be considered. Reconstruction of the comminution following open reduction with plate, or pin and cerclage wire fixation would be discouraged due to an extensive exposure and high potential for compromising vascularization. An interlocking nail should not be considered due to the small distal bone segment. MIPO should be considered, although the short distal bone segment would likely accommodate only two bone screws. External fixation with a bilateral, Type II, or hybrid ring fixator should be considered as they can be placed without disruption of the fracture and either technique will have adequate purchase of the distal segment.

Surgery Report
The patient was placed in the dorsal recumbent position with the limb suspended from the ceiling in a hanging limb technique so as to assist in fracture reduction. A preassembled hybrid fixator was placed on the limb and the limb resuspended. The hybrid fixator consisted of a 66 mm, 3.2 mm thick, partial ring attached to a 9.5 mm diameter 250 mm long connecting rod. Three olive wires were placed; two from medial, and one from lateral. The wires were tightened and secured on the opposite sides of the ring. A 3.2 mm end-threaded positive-profile fixator pin was inserted transversely into the proximal tibia and secured to the connecting rod. Limb alignment was visually confirmed. Two additional 3.2 mm pins were then placed from the medial connecting rod into the proximal 4th of the tibia. The third pin was angled somewhat proximally. A second connecting rod, attached to the proximal aspect of the medial connecting rod, coursed distally and laterally and was secured to the cranial-lateral aspect of the distal ring.

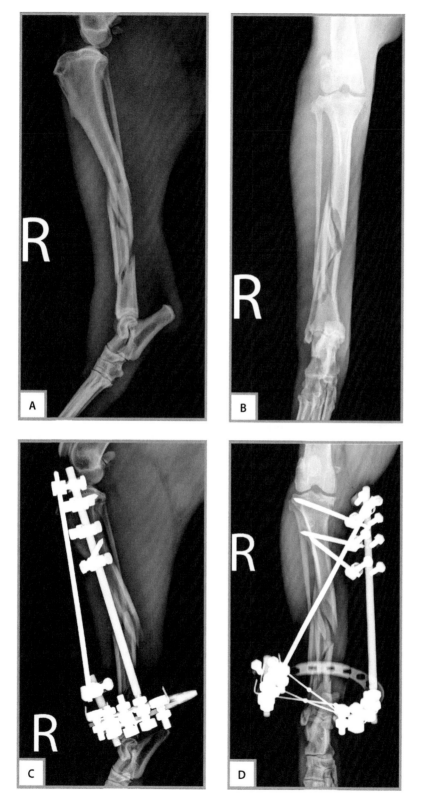

Figure 2.29 (A) Preoperative: lateral view; (B) Preoperative: cranial/caudal view; (C) Postoperative: lateral view; (D) Postoperative: cranial/caudal view.

(Continued)

Closed, Highly Comminuted Fracture of the Mid-to-Distal 4th of the Tibia *continued*

Postoperative Evaluation of Fracture Repair (Figures 2.29C–D)

Criteria	Assessment	Details
Alignment	Sufficient	There is slight lateral deviation of the distal tibia. Rotational alignment was adequate. There is marked caudal bowing of the fracture. Though some malalignment of the tibia can be tolerated in the cranial-to-caudal plane, this approaches an acceptable limit.
Apposition	Sufficient	There are large fracture gaps throughout the area of comminution, however, with the periosteum intact, healing is expected.
Apparatus	Sufficient	With three olive wires distally and three fixation pins proximal, together with interconnected constructs, the fixation is anticipated to provide adequate strength and stiffness. The 3rd fixation pin would be more structurally sound if it were closer to the fracture line and positioned perpendicular to the tibia.

Follow-up at 14 Weeks (Figures 2.29E–F)

Criteria	Assessment
Alignment	Unchanged
Apposition	Unchanged
Apparatus	The apparatus is unchanged in its construct. There is lucency around the three fixator pins in the proximal tibia; suggesting pin loosening. There is no lucency of the distal wires.
Activity	A recheck sooner than 14 weeks was recommended. Healing appears to be complete with smooth, remodeling callus throughout the fracture. There is caudal bowing of approximately 25 degrees at the mid-tibia. The patient was ambulating well and the fixator was removed with client instructions to slowly increase activity.

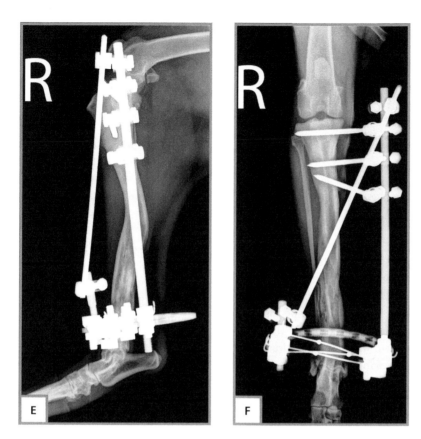

Figure 2.29 (Continued) (E) Follow-up at 14 Weeks: lateral view; (F) Follow-up at 14 Weeks: cranial/caudal view.

Closed, Comminuted Fracture of the Distal Tibia

Signalment and History
A 2-year-old, neutered, male Boxer weighing 30 kg sustained a left tibia fracture when his limb became entangled in a chain.

Patient Assessment
The young adult patient was in good health. Upon presentation the limb was swollen and was placed in a Robert Jones bandage.

Fracture Assessment
Closed, comminuted fracture of the distal two thirds of the tibia, minimally displaced and not over-riding (Figures 2.30A–B). This fracture was minimally displaced, and as such, the periosteum was presumed to be intact. Accordingly, the biological environment was optimal for fracture healing. The fibula was intact, which contributed to the stability of the fracture, and suggested that the tibia was never grossly displaced.

Options for Repair Methods
Because the fracture was not grossly displaced and had some inherent stability, splinting or casting could have been an appropriate choice. However, the fracture had long, oblique components and a large area of comminution throughout the distal two thirds of the tibia. Also, the distal extent of the fracture was very close to the joint. Internal fixation with a bone plate would not be favored, as the approach would have destabilized the fracture, compromised the microenvironment of the fracture, and six bone cortices could not have been engaged distally. A fixation with IM pins and cerclage wires, again, would require an extensive surgical exposure and the IM pins would not have countered bending forces. This would lead to the cerclage wires carrying excessive fixation reliance. External fixation of the tibia alone would only have allowed fixation of the distal segment with a ring or hybrid fixator. Although somewhat unconventional, a trans-tarsal external fixator would stabilize the fracture in medial-to-lateral bending, as well as torsion and would counter axial forces. Only small

cranial-to-caudal bending forces exist in the distal tibia.

Surgery Report
The patient was placed in the dorsal recumbent position with the affected limb in extension by suspension from the ceiling. The limb was left hanging throughout the procedure in 165 degrees of extension. All pins were positive-profile and were placed after pre-drilling the pin hole with a drill bit size being the minor diameter of the fixation pin. The first pin was a 4.0 mm positive-profile, center-threaded full pin placed across the proximal tibia just distal to the medial collateral ligament, exiting laterally; just cranial to the fibular head. The next pin was placed across the talus and calcaneus from medial-to-lateral. This was also a 4.0 mm full, center-threaded, positive-profile pin. In order to engage both the talus and calcaneus without placing the pin between the two bones, the drill hole was started slightly cranial and directed slightly caudal. Care was taken to not overheat the bone with the drill bit. Drill flutes were cleared often and the drill site was continuously lavaged. Medial and lateral 9.5 mm carbon-fiber connecting rods were placed and extended 2 cm distal to the fixator pin in the talus and calcaneus.

The next pins placed were 3.2 mm half-pins; placed into the distal row of tarsal bones. These connected to the distal connecting rods. Their placement was carefully planned so that they would not interfere with each other. Those prominences where the tarsus articulates with the 2nd and 5th tarsal bones were used as placement landmarks. These pins were either angled slightly or positioned with one directed slightly cranial and one slightly caudal. The first of these two pins placed was the lateral pin; introduced into the 4th tarsal bone. If possible, fixation pins placed in the distal row of tarsal bones should engage the 1st through 4th tarsal bones while fixation pins placed immediately proximal to that should engage both the central and 4th tarsal bones.

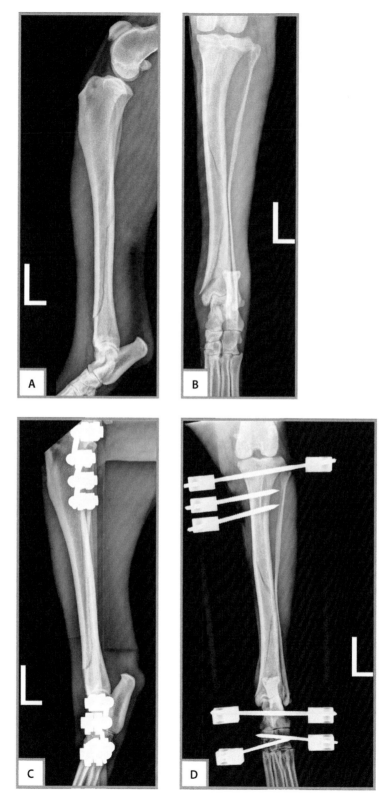

Figure 2.30 (A) Preoperative: lateral view; (B) Preoperative: cranial/caudal view; (C) Postoperative: lateral view; (D) Postoperative: cranial/caudal view.

(Continued)

Closed, Comminuted Fracture of the Distal Tibia *continued*

Placing a pin between the central tarsal bone and the 2nd and 3rd tarsal bones is to be avoided. The pins were angled slightly so that they engaged the distal two 'rows' of tarsal bones, thus avoiding the possibility of being placed between tarsal 'rows'. Two additional 3.2 mm half-pins were placed from the medial connecting rod in the proximal tibia, proximal to the fissure lines.

A soft padded bandage was applied for two days, after which the fixator frame was wrapped for the remainder of recovery.

Postoperative Evaluation of Fracture Repair (Figures 2.30C–D)

Criteria	Assessment	Details
Alignment	Optimal	The limb is in anatomic alignment.
Apposition	Good	The fracture gaps are more clearly seen as they appear to have widened compared to preoperative imaging. This likely occurred during fixation.
Apparatus	Good	The fixator frame contains two full-pins: one proximal and one distal to the fracture. This Type II construct has a mechanical advantage over a Type I construct consisting of only half-pins. There are a total of three pins above and three pins below the fracture, which is recommended. However, this is a trans-articular construct, where there is no support to the distal tibia which could move cranially and caudally. The fixation would be unstable if the fibula were not intact and the fracture displaced. Also, there is a large distance between the fixation pins. This allows a long lever arm between the pins and the fracture lines resulting in a comparatively less rigid fixation.

First Follow-up at 6 Weeks (Figures 2.30E–F)

Criteria	Assessment
Alignment	Unchanged
Apposition	Unchanged
Apparatus	Unchanged
Activity	There is minimal callus; suggesting adequate stability. The fracture lines are becoming more radio-opaque, validating that bone healing is occurring likely by a combination of primary and secondary bone union.

Final Follow-up at 9 Weeks (Figures 2.30G–H)

Criteria	Assessment
Alignment	Unchanged
Apposition	Unchanged
Apparatus	The proximal full pin has some lucency around it, suggesting pin loosening. It is common for this pin to become loose due to the micromovement of surrounding soft tissue (muscle).
Activity	Though fracture lines can still be şeen radiographically, the cortices are continuous medially, laterally, cranially and caudally which demonstrates adequate healing and that the fixator can be removed.

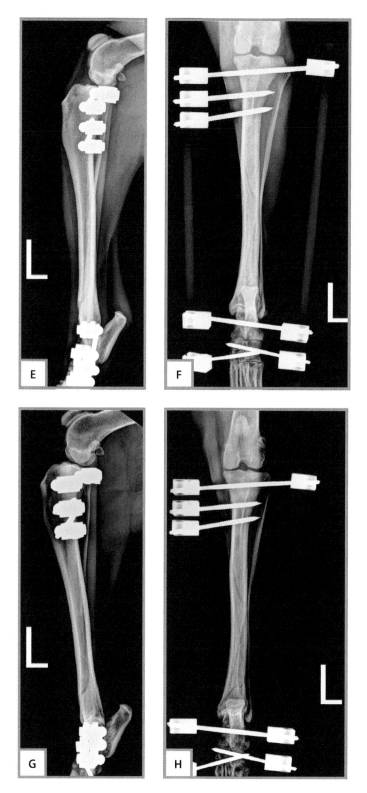

Figure 2.30 (Continued) (E) First Follow-up at 6 Weeks: lateral view; (F) First Follow-up at 6 Weeks: cranial/caudal view; (G) Second Follow-up at 9 Weeks: lateral view; (H) Second Follow-up at 9 Weeks: cranial/caudal view.

Closed, Salter I Fracture of the Left Distal Tibia

Signalment and History

A 1-year-old, intact, male Labrador Retriever weighing 35 kg sustained multiple fractures following a motor vehicle accident. These included a left femoral capital physeal fracture, left tibial fracture, right ilial shaft fracture and right acetabular fracture. Thoracic radiographs were unremarkable. Urinary bladder was intact. Pain sensation was elicited from the caudal limbs and tail, and the anus was intact.

Patient Assessment

This polytrauma case presents several challenges for surgical fixation and postoperative care. More robust fixation is required. Since there are bilateral fractures, the patient will not easily be able to guard its injuries. There will be an increased metabolic demand with this patient and increased risk of infection due to the multiple injuries and longer anticipated anesthesia time. The following is a discussion of the treatment of the tibial fracture only.

Fracture Assessment

Closed Salter I fracture of the left distal tibia, displaced laterally (Figures 2.31A–B).

Options for Repair Methods

Cross pinning or placing pins in Rush fashion are the most common methods of fixation. External coaptation might be considered if this was the only injury because it is minimally displaced. However, this would not be recommended in this patient due to the other musculoskeletal compromises.

Surgery Report

The patient was placed in the dorsal recumbent position and approaches to both the medial and lateral malleoli were performed. The fracture was reduced with the assistance of pointed reduction forceps. Location of the talocrural joint was determined using a 25 gauge needle. Two 1.6 mm (14 gauge) Kirschner wires were driven across the physis into the metaphysis at 45 degree angles from the distal aspect of each malleoli. The approach was closed routinely.

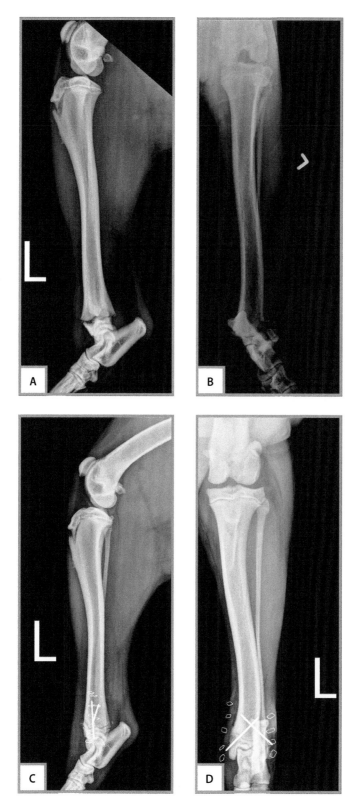

Figure 2.31 (A) Preoperative: lateral view; (B) Preoperative: cranial/caudal view; (C) Postoperative: lateral view; (D) Postoperative: cranial/caudal view.

(Continued)

Closed, Salter I Fracture of the Left Distal Tibia *continued*

Postoperative Evaluation of Fracture Repair (Figures 2.31C–D)

Criteria	Assessment	Details
Alignment	Optimal	The fracture is anatomically reduced.
Apposition	Optimal	The physis appears normal in width.
Apparatus	Optimal	The Kirschner wires were small, but needed to be large enough to engage the small malleoli, while small enough to avoid malleoli fracturing. Although robust fixation would typically be needed for this type of fracture, the patient's relative immobilization due to multiple fractures renders this repair sufficient. Compressive forces across the fracture from the pull of the common calcaneal tendon will be present during ambulation. Although there will be shear forces on the fracture line, the pins are able to counter these forces. There would not be excessive bending forces on the pins since they are bilateral. Bending of the limb would result primarily in shear forces on this fracture.

Follow-up at 7 Weeks (Figures 2.31E–F)

Criteria	Assessment
Alignment	Unchanged
Apposition	Unchanged
Apparatus	Unchanged
Activity	There is minimal callus, suggesting little motion during healing. The physis is no longer visible, indicating a healed fracture.

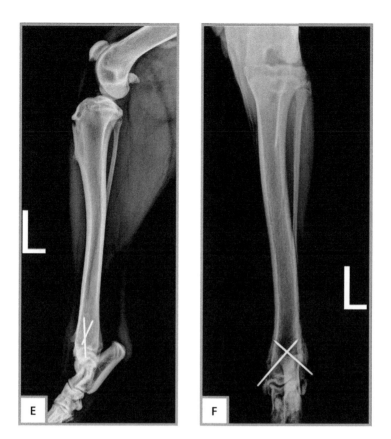

Figure 2.31 (Continued) (E) Follow-up at 7 Weeks: lateral view; (F) Follow-up at 7 Weeks: cranial/caudal view.

Closed, Comminuted Fracture of the Right Central Calcaneus

Signalment and History
A 7-year-old, neutered, male Greyhound weighing 43 kg sustained a tarsal fracture while racing around a corner. The patient was in good health and physical examination revealed no abnormalities other than the rear limb injury.

Patient Assessment
Racing greyhounds place considerable force on the tarsus as evident by the high incidence of right, central, tarsal bone fractures observed.

Fracture Assessment
Closed, comminuted fracture of the right central calcaneus (Figures 2.32A–B).

Options for Repair Methods
Especially in the greyhound, the tarsus is an area of scant soft tissue coverage and therefore low biological activity. This is also bone that is subject to very large forces due to the weight-bearing, lever arm of the distal limb and short length of the calcaneus. This amplifies forces on the calcaneus. Because of proximity to the joint and low biological activity, fixation techniques yielding primary bone union should be chosen; specifically an open reduction with internal plate fixation. Because of the large forces involved, implant constructs should be chosen that allow load-sharing rather than load solely born by the implant. In addition, the use of multiple implants should be considered to increase the AMI of the construct. Plate fixation with interfragmentary screws if appropriate should be chosen. External support alone, pin and wire fixation or external fixators should not be used solely as primary repair.

Surgery Report
The patient was placed in the left lateral recumbent position. A lateral approach to the calcaneus and plantar aspects of the tarsal bones was performed, while Gelpi retractors were used to maintain retraction. Pointed reduction forceps were placed on the calcaneal tuber in a mediolateral direction to apply caudal-to-distal traction to the body of the calcaneus. A second pointed reduction forcep was placed from the central tarsal bone cranially to the 4th tarsal bone caudally so as to aid in reduction of the distal intertarsal joint. A 9-hole, 2.4 mm locking plate was placed along the caudolateral length of the calcaneus, subtending the base of the intertarsal joint. Five screws were applied in sequence from proximal-to-distal, leaving screw holes 3–6 open. Fracture fragments adjacent to the sustantaculum tali at the base of the calcaneus were reduced with Freer elevator manipulation. A 4-hole, 2.0 mm locking plate was placed across a fracture at the base of the calcaneal tuber and all screw holes were filled. A 3-hole 2.0 mm locking plate was placed across yet another fracture line in the calcaneus located just proximal to the proximal intertarsal joint, leaving the middle screw hole empty. The approach was closed routinely, and the patient was placed in a splint for 6 weeks.

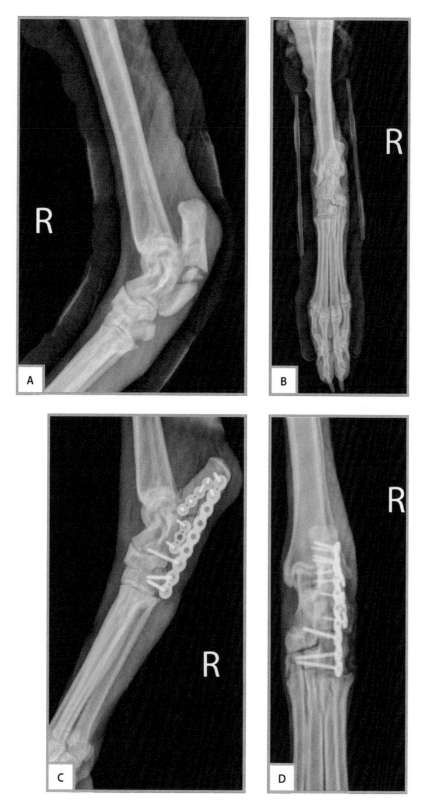

Figure 2.32 (A) Preoperative: lateral view; (B) Preoperative: dorsalplantar view; (C) Postoperative: lateral view; (D) Postoperative: dorsalplantar view.

(Continued)

Closed, Comminuted Fracture of the Right Central Calcaneus *continued*

Postoperative Evaluation of Fracture Repair (Figures 2.32C–D)

Criteria	Assessment	Details
Alignment	Optimal	The fracture is anatomically reduced to re-establish alignment.
Apposition	Sufficient	Though the fracture has been anatomically reconstructed, fracture lines are still visible.
Apparatus	Good	A locking plate system was chosen, although it may have been preferable to choose DCPs to achieve interfragmentary compression. The 2.4 mm plate has only two screws engaging the calcaneous and four open screw holes due to the configuration of comminution. The two additional 2.0 mm plates assist in stabilizing the additional fractures, and also reduce load on the 2.4 mm plate by increasing the AMI of the bone/implant construct. Still, the 2.4 mm plate and two 2.0 mm plates are rather small considering those forces on the calcaneus. Accordingly, additional external support would be advised to protect the construct.

Follow-up at 11 Weeks (Figures 2.32E–F)

Criteria	Assessment
Alignment	Unchanged
Apposition	Unchanged
Apparatus	Unchanged
Activity	Fracture lines observable in the postoperative radiographs have resolved without noticeable callus; suggesting primary bone union of the callus and healing. The patient was slowly returned to activity. The tarsus is considered a rather 'non-forgiving' joint and osteoarthritis is likely.

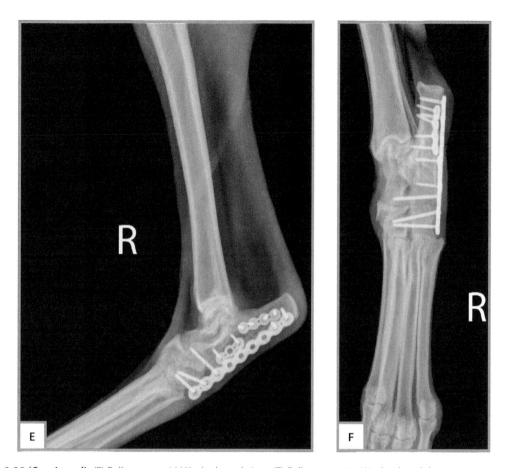

Figure 2.32 (Continued) (E) Follow-up at 11 Weeks: lateral view; (F) Follow-up at 11 Weeks: dorsalplantar view.

Closed, Transverse Fracture of the Proximal Calcaneus

Signalment and History
A 6-month-old, intact, male Boston Terrier weighing 5.5 kg sustained a calcaneus fracture after falling down a flight of stairs.

Patient Assessment
No other injuries were sustained. The patient is young with good healing potential.

Fracture Assessment
Closed, transverse fracture of the proximal calcaneus, with the proximal bone segment displaced proximally and medially 0.5 mm (Figures 2.33A–B). Calcaneal fractures are difficult to stabilize and slow to heal. This patient is juvenile with robust healing potential. However, this area is compromised biologically, with low blood supply, and mechanically, with large distractive forces from the common calcaneal tendon. In addition, there is less than 1 cm length of proximal calcaneus for implant purchase, making rigid fixation difficult. Comminuted calcaneal fractures are especially difficult to repair and are associated with a high rate of failure.

Options for Repair Methods
External support would not be appropriate. As the calcaneus is under tension, fixation must counter the large pull of the common calcaneal tendon. Tension band fixation has been described; however, it can be difficult to place Kirschner wires or small pins in the hard bone of the calcaneous. Also, a tension band should be placed under the superficial digital flexor and in such a fashion that the fracture is stable with the tension band providing a counter to traction on the plantar aspect of the calcaneus. Tension banding takes advantage of two forces (typically, that of a tendon and that of the cerclage wire) yielding a compressive summation force across a fracture line. This case does not fit that model. Failure with tension banding in this type of fracture is not uncommon.

If there is sufficient bone, then plate fixation can be attempted. Rarely can three screws be placed in the proximally avulsed bone segment. Plate fixation should be with the plate placed as caudally as possible to counter the tensile force from the pull of the calcaneal tendon. However, the calcaneus is narrow and the superficial digital flexor runs over this surface. For this reason, plates are placed laterally but as caudal as possible.

Surgery Report
The patient was placed in dorsal recumbency and an approach to the calcaneus was performed. The fracture was reduced and a 5-hole, locking 2.7 mm T-plate was applied. The plate was contoured to the bone and a screw placed in the second, more plantar hole of the T-section of the plate. This was to ensure solid bone stock. A second screw was then placed in screw hole 4, second from the distal end of the plate. The first screw was then placed, angling slightly distal and caudal so as to again purchase as much bone as possible. A screw was then placed in screw hole 5. Screw hole 3 was left open because screw placement would have entered the fracture line. The approach was closed routinely. The limb was placed in extension with a lateral splint for the duration of healing.

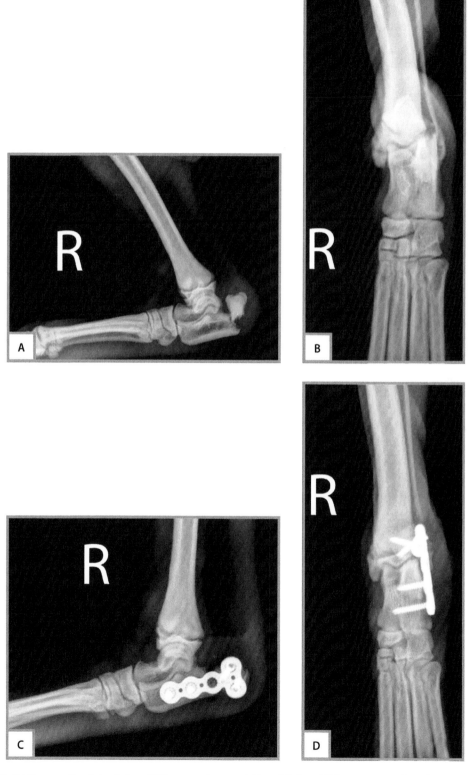

Figure 2.33 (A) Preoperative: lateral view; (B) Preoperative: cranial/caudal view; (C) Postoperative: lateral view; (D) Postoperative: cranial/caudal view.

(Continued)

Closed, Transverse Fracture of the Proximal Calcaneus *continued*

Postoperative Evaluation of Fracture Repair (Figures 2.33C–D)

Criteria	Assessment	Details
Alignment	Optimal	The fracture is anatomically reduced.
Apposition	Good	The fracture line is still visible radiographically, albeit small.
Apparatus	Sufficient	There are limits to fixation options due to the fracture configurations and available instrumentation. A locking plate was chosen. This should provide better security of the small avulsed segment, as the screw is angle-stable and not reliant on the holding power of the screw treads to grasp the segment. However, locking plates cannot provide compression of the fracture. The small fracture segment allowed placement of only two screws. Two screws engaged the calcaneus distally. This implant is available only in a 5-hole configuration. Screw hole 3 adjacent to the T-section was left open due to it being close to the fracture line. This presents a weak, but unavoidable, area of the fixation. External support should always be an accessory accommodation with calcaneal fractures; therefore, the fixation was supported with a splint.

First Follow-up at 5 Weeks (Figures 2.33E–F)

Criteria	Assessment
Alignment	Unchanged
Apposition	Unchanged
Apparatus	Unchanged
Activity	Due to overlying implant and anatomic structures, the fracture line cannot be clearly visualized on the lateral view. On the cranial/caudal view the fracture line appears to be healing. The splint was removed and strict exercise restriction was imposed.

Final Follow-up at 8 Weeks (Figures 2.33G–H)

Criteria	Assessment
Alignment	Unchanged
Apposition	Unchanged
Apparatus	Unchanged
Activity	The fracture line appears healed. The patient was slowly returned to normal activity.

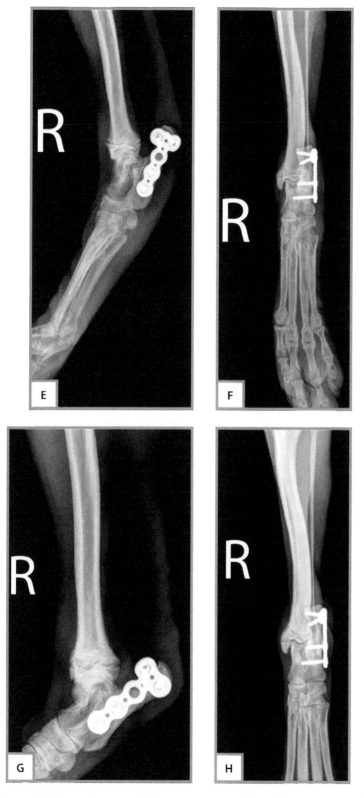

Figure 2.33 (Continued) (E) First Follow-up at 5 Weeks: lateral view; (F) First Follow-up at 5 Weeks: cranial/caudal view; (G) Final Follow-up at 8 Weeks: lateral view; (H) Final Follow-up at 8 Weeks: cranial/caudal view.

Closed, Transverse Fracture of the Tibial Tarsal Bone

Signalment and History
A 4-year-old, neutered, male West Highland White Terrier weighing 9 kg sustained an injury of the left caudal limb after jumping from a slow moving vehicle. The patient was not weight-bearing and radiographs taken soon after the injury did not reveal skeletal abnormalities.

Patient Assessment
The patient presented 7 weeks following the initial injury for intermittent non-weight bearing of the left caudal limb. There was modest muscle atrophy and crepitation was elicited on palpation of the left talocrural joint. The patient was in good condition. Additional radiographs were obtained.

Fracture Assessment
Closed, transverse fracture of the tibial tarsal bone between the trochlea and head. The fracture was non-displaced. Early osteoarthritis was noted (Figures 2.34A–B).

Options for Repair Methods
The fracture was in an area of probable low vascularity and metabolic activity. In addition, the fracture was 7 weeks old and the patient had been ambulating to some degree, thereby wearing the fracture ends. The fracture would need open reduction and rigid internal fixation with compression to achieve primary boney union. External support using splints or casts would be unlikely to achieve union. Lag screw fixation would achieve compression. Accurately placing a lag screw from a caudal approach would be difficult and would require an arthrotomy to ensure reduction and proper screw placement.

Lagging through the trochlea would require creating a cartilage defect in order to counter-sink the head of the screw. Metabolic activity of this tarsal bone is low, and an autogenous cancellous bone graft may interfere with compression of the lag screw as well as introduce 'bone debris' into the joint. Demineralized bone matrix is commercially available in a consistency that could stimulate biological activity yet still allow compression.

Surgery Report
An approach to the tarsocrural joint by osteotomy of the medial malleolus was performed. Prior to performing the osteotomy a drill hole was made using a 1.5 mm drill bit in anticipation of replacing the malleolus. The hole was then measured for depth and tapped for a 2.0 mm screw. The fracture was reduced and a 1.1 mm drill bit used to drill a hole from the trochlea into the neck of the tibial tarsal bone followed by measuring and tapping. A 1.5 mm drill bit was then used to over-drill the trochlea, followed with a 2.0 mm drill bit to countersink the head of a positioned 1.5 mm screw. This sequencing left the head of the inserted screw 1 mm below the articular surface. A small amount of demineralized bone matrix combined with biphasic calcium phosphate and fine mineralized cancellous chips (Fusion Xpress, Veterinary Transplant Services, Inc., Kent, WA) was placed on the fracture surfaces prior to tightening the screw. The malleolus was replaced and compressed with pointed bone-holding forceps. The screw was placed without over-drilling the malleolus for preservation of as much bone as possible. Closure was routine.

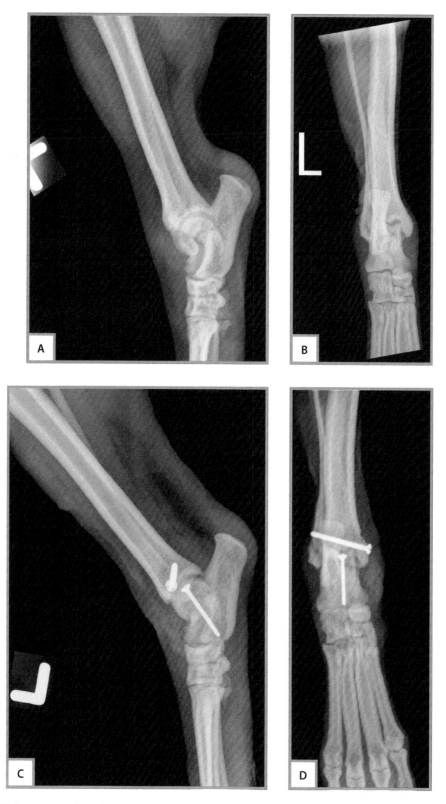

Figure 2.34 (A) Preoperative: lateral view; (B) Preoperative: dorsalplantar view; (C) Postoperative: lateral view; (D) Postoperative: dorsalplantar view.

(Continued)

Closed, Transverse Fracture of the Tibial Tarsal Bone *continued*

Postoperative Evaluation of Fracture Repair (Figures 2.34C–D)

Criteria	Assessment	Details
Alignment	Optimal	The fracture is anatomically reduced.
Apposition	Good	The fracture line was still visible.
Apparatus	Sufficient	Only a 1.5 mm screw was used for fixation of this fracture. The minor diameter of this screw was less than 1.1 mm. The AMI would be very small. Any motion of this segment could result in cyclic loading of the implant and screw breakage.

First Follow-up at 6 Weeks (Figures 2.34E–F)

Criteria	Assessment
Alignment	Unchanged
Apposition	Unchanged
Apparatus	Unchanged
Activity	Good; no callus could be visualized. The fracture lines were less apparent.

Final Follow-up at 8 Weeks (Figures 2.34G–H)

Criteria	Assessment
Alignment	Unchanged
Apposition	Unchanged
Apparatus	Unchanged
Activity	Good; fracture lines are not discernible. Osteoarthritis does not appear to have progressed from preoperative imaging. The patient was slowly returned to normal activity.

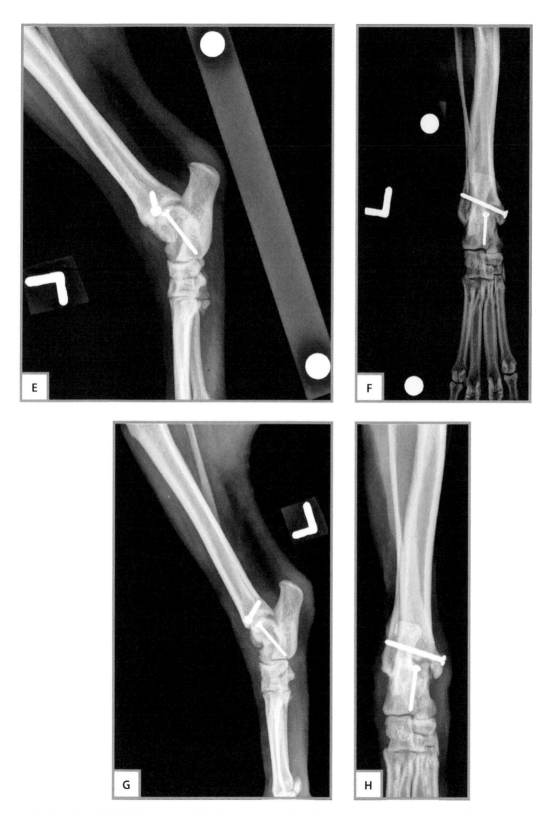

Figure 2.34 (Continued) (E) Follow-up at 6 Weeks: lateral view; (F) Follow-up at 6 Weeks: dorsalplantar view; (G) Follow-up at 8 Weeks: lateral view; (H) Follow-up at 8 Weeks: dorsalplantar view.

Bibliographic References

1. Wheeless CR, 'Bone and fracture healing', in *Wheeless' textbook of orthopaedics* edited by Wheeless CR, Brooklandville, Data Trace Internet Publishing, LLC, (2015) (http://www.wheelessonline.com/ortho/8342, accessed April 2016).

2. Giannoudis PV, Einhorn TA and Marsh D, 'Fracture healing: the diamond concept', *Injury* 38 Suppl 4 (2007):S3–6.

3. Giannoudis PV, Einhorn TA and Marsh D, 'Fracture healing: a harmony of optimal biology and optimal fixation?' *Injury* 38 Suppl 4 (2007):S1–2.

4. Perren SM, 'Evolution of the internal fixation of long bone fractures. The scientific basis of biological internal fixation: choosing a new balance between stability and biology', *J Bone Joint Surg Br* 84 (2002):1093–1110.

5. Welch JA, Boudrieau RJ, DeJardin LM and Spodnick GJ, 'The intraosseous blood supply of the canine radius: implications for healing of distal fractures in small dogs', *Vet Surg* 26 (1997):57–61.

6. Dudley M, Johnson AL, Olmstead M, Smith CW, Schaeffler DJ and Abbuehl U, 'Open reduction and bone plate stabilization, compared with closed reduction and external fixation, for treatment of comminuted tibial fractures: 47 cases (1980–1995) in dogs', *J Am Vet Med Assoc* 211 (1997):1008–1012.

7. Gruber R, Koch H, Doll BA, Tegtmeier F, Einhorn TA and Hollinger JO, 'Fracture healing in the elderly patient', *Exp Gerontol* 41 (2006):1080–1093.

8. Kraus KH, Toombs JP and Ness MG, 'External fixation in small animal practice', (2003) Boston, Wiley-Blackwell.

9. Miller EI, Acquaviva AE, Eisenmann DJ, Stone RT and Kraus KH, 'Perpendicular pull-out force of locking versus non-locking plates in thin cortical bone using a canine mandibular ramus model', *Vet Surg* 40 (2011):870–874.

10. Gustilo RB and Anderson JT, 'JSBS classics. Prevention of infection in the treatment of one thousand and twenty-five open fractures of long bones. Retrospective and prospective analyses', *J Bone Joint Surg Am* 84-A (2002):682.

11. Anderson JT, Gustilo RB, 'Immediate internal fixation in open fractures', *Orthop Clin North Am* 11 (1980):569–578.

12. Wheeless CR, 'Open Fractures' in *Wheeless' Textbook of Orthopedics* edited by Wheeless CR. Brooklandville, Data Trace Internet Publishing, LLC, (2015) (http://www.wheelessonline.com/ortho/open_fractures, accessed April 2016).

13. Mercer University School of Medicine 'Fire Arms Tutorial Ballistics' in *The Internet Pathology Laboratory* hosted by The University of Utah, Eccles Health Sciences Library (2015) (http://library.med.utah.edu/WebPath/TUTORIAL/GUNS/GUNINTRO.html, accessed April 2016).

14. Augat P, Burger J, Schorlemmer S, Henke T, Peraus M and Claes L, 'Shear movement at the fracture site delays healing in a diaphyseal fracture model' *J Orthop Res* 21 (2003):1011–1017.

15. Beer FP, Johnston ER, DeWolf JT and Mazurek DF *Mechanics of Materials* (7th edition). New York, McGraw Hill Education, (2014).

16. Kerwin SC 'Fixation with pins and wires; Application of cerclage and hemi-cerclage wires', in *Current techniques in small animal surgery* (5th edition) edited by Bojrab MJ, WY, Teton NewMedia, (2014).

17. Roe SC, 'Evaluation of tension obtained by use of three knots for tying cerclage wires by surgeons of various abilities and experience', *J Am Vet Med Assoc* 220 (2002):334–336.

18. Roe SC, 'Mechanical characteristics and comparisons of cerclage wires: introduction of the double-wrap and loop/twist tying methods', *Vet Surg* 26 (1997):310–316.

19. Chapman MW, 'The effect of reamed and non-reamed intramedullary nailing on fracture healing', *Clin Orthop Relat Res* 355 Suppl (1998):S230-S238.

20. Sissener TR, Jones E and Langley-Hobbs SJ, 'Effects of three intramedullary pinning techniques on pin location and articular damage in the canine humerus', *Vet Comp Orthop Traumatol* 18(2005):153–156.

21. Dallman MJ, Martin RA, Self BP and Grant JW, 'Rotational strength of double-pinning techniques in repair of transverse fractures in femurs of dogs', *Am J Vet Res* 51 (1990):123–127.

22. Dejardin LM, Cabassu JB, Guillou RP, Villwock M, Guiot LP and Haut RC, 'In vivo biomechanical evaluation of a novel angle-stable interlocking nail design in a canine tibial fracture model', *Vet Surg* 43 (2014):271–281.

23. Dejardin LM, Lansdowne JL, Sinnott MT, Sidebotham CG and Haut RC, 'In vitro mechanical evaluation of torsional loading in simulated canine tibiae for a novel hourglass-shaped interlocking nail with a self-tapping tapered locking design', *Am J Vet Res* 67 (2006):678–685.

24. Lansdowne JL, Sinnott MT, Dejardin LM, Ting D and Haut RC, 'In vitro mechanical comparison of screwed, bolted, and novel interlocking nail systems to buttress plate fixation in torsion and mediolateral bending', *Vet Surg* 36 (2007):368–377.

25. Hupel TM, Aksenov SA, Schemitsch EH, 'Effect of limited and standard reaming on cortical bone blood flow and early strength of union following segmental fracture', *J Orthop Trauma* 12 (1998):400–406.

26. Wheeless CR, 'Theory of dynamic compression plates' in *Wheeless' Textbook of Orthopedics* edited by Wheeless CR. Brooklandville, Data Trace Internet Publishing, LLC, (2015) (http://www.wheelessonline.com/ortho/theory_of_dynamic_compression_plates, accessed April 2016).

27. Kraus KH, Kadiyala S, Wotton H, Kruth A, Shea M, Hannan M, Hayes WC, Kirker-Head CA and Bruder S, 'Critically sized osteo-periosteal femoral defects: a dog model', *J Invest Surg* 12 (1999):115–124.

28. Demianiuk RM, Benamou J, Rutherford S, Beckett S, Ness MG and Dejardin LM, 'Effect of screw type and distribution on the torsional stability of 3.5 mm string of pearls locking plate constructs', *Vet Surg* 44 (2015):119–125.

29. Reems MR, Beale BS and Hulse DA, 'Use of a plate-rod construct and principles of biological osteosynthesis for repair of diaphyseal fractures in dogs and cats: 47 cases (1994–2001)', *J Am Vet Med Assoc* 223 (2003):330–335.

30. Acquaviva AE, Miller EI, Eisenmann DJ, Stone RT and Kraus KH, 'Biomechanical testing of locking and non-locking plates in the canine scapula', *J Am Anim Hosp Assoc* 48 (2012):372–378.

31. Gardner MJ, Brophy RH, Campbell D, Mahajan A, Wright TM, Helfet DL and Lorich DG, 'The mechanical behavior of locking compression plates compared with dynamic compression plates in a cadaver radius model', *J Orthop Trauma* 19 (2005):597–603.

32. Tejwani NC and Wolinsky P, 'The changing face of orthopaedic trauma: locked plating and minimally invasive techniques', *Instr Course Lect* 57 (2008):3–9.

33. Strauss EJ, Schwarzkopf R, Kummer F and Egol KA, 'The current status of locked plating: the good, the bad, and the ugly', *J Orthop Trauma* 22 (2008):479–486.

34. Boero Baroncelli A, Reif U, Bignardi C and Peirone B, 'Effect of screw insertion torque on push-out and cantilever bending properties of five different angle-stable systems', *Vet Surg* 42 (2013):308–315.

35. Hudson CC, Pozzi A and Lewis DD, 'Minimally invasive plate osteosynthesis: applications and techniques in dogs and cats', *Vet Comp Orthop Traumatol*, 22 (2009):175–182.

36. Perren SM, 'The technology of minimally invasive percutaneous osteosynthesis (MIPO)', *Injury* 33 Suppl 1 (2002):VI–VII.

37. Schmokel HG, Stein S, Radke H, Hurter K and Schawalder P, 'Treatment of tibial fractures with plates using minimally invasive percutaneous osteosynthesis in dogs and cats', *J Small Anim Pract* 48 (2007):157–160.

38. White DT, Bronson DG and Welch RD, 'A mechanical comparison of veterinary linear external fixation systems', *Vet Surg* 32 (2003):507–514.

39. Kraus KH, Wotton HM, Boudrieau RJ, Schwarz L, Diamond D and Minihan A, 'Type-II external fixation, using new clamps and positive-profile threaded pins, for treatment of fractures of the radius and tibia in dogs', *J Am Vet Med Assoc* 212 (1998):1267–1270.

40. Gorman SC, Kraus KH, Keating JH, Tidwell AS, Rand WM, Parkington JD and Boudrieau RJ, 'In vivo axial dynamization of canine tibial fractures using the Securos external skeletal fixation system', *Vet Comp Orthop Traumatol* 18 (2005):199–207.

41. Dismukes DI, Fox DB, Tomlinson JL and Essman SC, 'Use of radiographic measures and three-dimensional computed tomographic imaging in surgical correction of an antebrachial deformity in a dog', *J Am Vet Med Assoc* 232 (2008):68–73.

42. Blaeser LL, Gallagher JG, and Boudrieau RJ, 'Treatment of biologically inactive nonunions by a limited en bloc ostectomy and compression plate fixation: a review of 17 cases', *Vet Surg* 32 (2003):91–100.

43. Tomlinson J, 'Minimally invasive repair of sacroiliac luxation in small animals', *Vet Clin North Am Small Anim Pract* 42 (2012):1069–1077.

44. Bowlt KL and Shales CJ, 'Canine sacroiliac luxation: anatomic study of the craniocaudal articular surface angulation of the sacrum to define a safe corridor in the dorsal plan for placement of screws used for fixation in lag fashion', *Vet Surg* 40 (2011):22–26.

Index

Printed and bound by CPI Group (UK) Ltd, Croydon, CR0 4YY

24/10/2024

01778285-0014